Graceful Aging: Chair Yoga for Seniors Over 60

Susanne J. Katts

Legal Disclaimer
The information contained in this book is for educational and informational purposes only and is not intended as medical advice. The author, Susanne J. Katts, is not a licensed medical professional, and the content should not be used to diagnose, treat, or replace professional medical guidance. Always consult with a qualified healthcare provider before beginning any exercise program, including chair yoga, especially if you have any pre-existing medical conditions or concerns.

The author and publisher disclaim any liability for any adverse effects arising directly or indirectly from the use of the information contained in this book. The exercises and recommendations presented herein are meant to be implemented safely, but individual results may vary. Readers assume full responsibility for their safety and well-being.

By using this book, you acknowledge and agree to the terms and conditions of this disclaimer. If you do not agree with these terms, please refrain from using the information provided in this book.

Trademarks

"Graceful Aging: Chair Yoga for Seniors Over 60"

Preface

Welcome to Graceful Aging: Chair Yoga for Seniors Over 60. This book is born out of a deep passion for empowering seniors to live healthier, happier, and more active lives. As we age, maintaining physical fitness, mental clarity, and emotional well-being becomes increasingly important, and chair yoga offers a uniquely accessible path to achieving these goals.

Chair yoga is not just about stretching and poses; it is a holistic practice that integrates the body, mind, and spirit. It provides a safe and adaptable way for seniors to experience the profound benefits of yoga, regardless of physical limitations. Whether you are new to yoga or have practiced for years, this book is designed to meet you where you are and help you build a sustainable and enjoyable practice.

In my years of teaching yoga, I have seen firsthand the incredible transformations that occur when seniors incorporate chair yoga into their daily routines. I have witnessed increased flexibility, strength, and balance, but perhaps more importantly, I have seen the joy, confidence, and community that yoga fosters. These experiences have inspired me to compile this comprehensive guide, with the hope that it will reach and benefit even more people.

This book is structured to be your companion on this journey. It begins with foundational knowledge, providing a clear understanding of what chair yoga is, its history, and its myriad benefits. From there, you will find practical advice on getting started safely, including consulting your doctor and setting up a conducive space for practice. The heart of the book lies in the detailed instructions for various routines, from beginner to advanced, tailored to specific health concerns and needs.

Beyond the physical practice, I have included chapters on enhancing your yoga journey with mindfulness, proper nutrition, and maintaining consistency. You will also find resources for connecting with others, finding classes, and accessing further reading to deepen your knowledge. Real-life stories and testimonials offer inspiration and demonstrate the real-world impact of chair yoga.

As you embark on this journey, I encourage you to approach it with an open heart and a willingness to explore and enjoy each step. Yoga is not a destination but a lifelong practice that evolves with you. May this book serve as a guide and a source of inspiration, helping you to embrace the many benefits of chair yoga and to age gracefully, with strength and serenity.

Thank you for allowing me to be a part of your yoga journey. I am honored to share this practice with you and excited for the positive changes it will bring to your life.

Namaste,
Susanne J. Katts

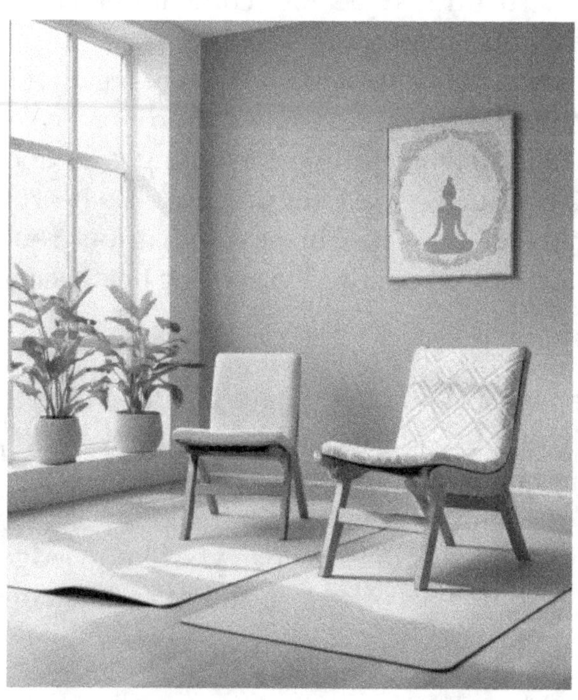

Introduction

Welcome to Graceful Aging: Chair Yoga for Seniors Over 60. This book is your gateway to discovering the transformative benefits of yoga, with a special focus on chair yoga designed specifically for seniors. As we age, maintaining physical health, mental clarity, and emotional well-being becomes increasingly important. Chair yoga offers a safe, accessible, and effective way to achieve these goals, regardless of your fitness level or physical limitations.

Chair yoga is a unique form of yoga that adapts traditional poses to be performed while seated or using a chair for support. This adaptation makes yoga more accessible to seniors, providing all the benefits of traditional yoga without the need to get down on the floor. Through gentle movements, mindful breathing, and relaxation techniques, chair yoga helps improve flexibility, strength, balance, and mental focus.

In this book, you will find everything you need to begin and sustain a rewarding chair yoga practice. We start by explaining why chair yoga is particularly suitable for seniors, highlighting its safety, accessibility, and numerous health benefits. From there, we guide you step-by-step through the basics, offering detailed instructions for various poses, breathing techniques, and routines tailored to different levels of experience and specific health concerns.

Whether you are new to yoga or looking to adapt your practice to better suit your needs, this book is designed to support you every step of the way. We provide practical advice on how to get started, including consulting your doctor, choosing the right chair, and setting up a comfortable practice space. Additionally, we offer tips for enhancing your practice with mindfulness, proper nutrition, and maintaining consistency.

Throughout the book, you will find real-life stories and testimonials from seniors who have experienced the positive impacts of chair yoga, providing inspiration and motivation. We also include a wealth of resources for further reading, finding classes, and connecting with supportive communities.

Embark on this journey with an open heart and a willingness to explore the many benefits of chair yoga. May this practice bring you increased vitality, serenity, and joy as you embrace the graceful process of aging.

Namaste,

Susanne J. Katts

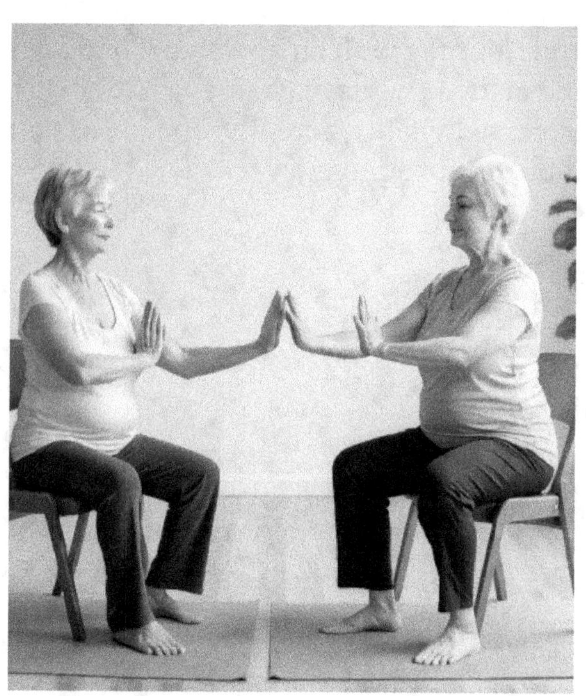

Chapter 2: Why Chair Yoga?

Chair yoga is an ideal form of exercise for seniors, offering a gentle yet effective way to improve physical health, mental clarity, and emotional well-being. Here's why chair yoga is particularly suitable for seniors:

Safety
Reduced Risk of Injury: Traditional yoga poses can sometimes be challenging for seniors, especially those with limited mobility or balance issues. Chair yoga modifies these poses to be performed while seated or using a chair for support, significantly reducing the risk of falls and injuries.

Gentle Movements: Chair yoga emphasizes slow, controlled movements that are easy on the joints and muscles. This is particularly beneficial for seniors with arthritis or other chronic conditions that make high-impact activities uncomfortable or unsafe.

Accessible for All Fitness Levels: Whether you are new to exercise or a seasoned yogi, chair yoga offers modifications that can be tailored to individual capabilities. This inclusivity ensures that everyone can participate and benefit, regardless of their physical condition.

Accessibility
Convenient and Versatile: Chair yoga can be practiced almost anywhere, from your living room to a community center, requiring only a sturdy chair. This convenience eliminates the need for special equipment or a yoga mat, making it easy to incorporate into daily routines.

Adaptable for Various Conditions: Chair yoga can be adapted to accommodate a wide range of health conditions and physical limitations. Whether you are dealing with mobility issues, recovering from surgery, or managing a chronic illness, chair yoga offers poses and routines that can be modified to meet your specific needs.

Low-Cost: Compared to other fitness programs that may require costly memberships or equipment, chair yoga is a low-cost option. A simple chair and minimal props like yoga straps or blocks are often all that's needed, making it an affordable way to stay active.

Benefits
Physical Benefits:

Improved Flexibility: Regular practice of chair yoga helps maintain and improve flexibility, which is crucial for performing daily activities with ease.
Increased Strength: Even gentle poses can help build muscle strength, particularly in the core, legs, and arms, supporting better posture and balance.
Enhanced Balance and Stability: Chair yoga includes exercises that enhance balance and coordination, reducing the risk of falls—a common concern for seniors.
Pain Management: The gentle stretching and strengthening exercises can alleviate chronic pain, particularly in the back, joints, and muscles.
Mental Benefits:

Stress Reduction: Chair yoga incorporates breathing exercises and mindfulness techniques that help reduce stress and promote relaxation.
Improved Mental Clarity: Regular practice can enhance concentration and cognitive function, helping to maintain mental sharpness.

Emotional Well-being: The meditative aspects of chair yoga encourage a sense of calm and emotional stability, reducing symptoms of anxiety and depression.
Social and Emotional Benefits:

Community Building: Participating in chair yoga classes can provide social interaction, fostering a sense of community and reducing feelings of isolation.
Emotional Support: Sharing the practice with others can offer emotional support and encouragement, enhancing overall well-being.
Self-Confidence: Mastering new poses and routines can boost self-esteem and confidence, empowering seniors to take charge of their health.
Chair yoga is a safe, accessible, and beneficial practice that can significantly enhance the quality of life for seniors. By integrating gentle movements, mindful breathing, and relaxation techniques, chair yoga provides a holistic approach to maintaining physical health, mental clarity, and emotional well-being. Embrace chair yoga as a means to age gracefully, with strength, balance, and peace.

Detailed Responses to Reader Questions

1. How do I get started with chair yoga?

What type of chair should I use?

Choose a sturdy, armless chair with a flat seat and a straight back. The chair should be stable and not have wheels. A dining chair or a folding chair works well.

Are there any specific accessories or props that are recommended for beginners?

Useful props include yoga straps (or a belt/towel), yoga blocks, and a cushion or blanket for added comfort and support.

2. What precautions should I take before starting chair yoga?

Do I need to consult my doctor before beginning?

Yes, it is always advisable to consult with your healthcare provider before starting any new exercise program, especially if you have pre-existing health conditions.

What are the signs that I might be pushing myself too hard?

Signs include sharp pain, dizziness, shortness of breath, and excessive fatigue. Listen to your body and avoid any movements that cause discomfort.

3. How often should I practice chair yoga to see benefits?

Is there an optimal frequency or duration for each session?

Aim to practice chair yoga 3-5 times a week. Each session can range from 15 to 45 minutes, depending on your comfort level and schedule.

4. Are there specific routines for particular health conditions?

What poses or routines are best for managing arthritis, back pain, or osteoporosis?

For arthritis, gentle stretches and movements that enhance joint mobility are beneficial.

For back pain, focus on strengthening and stretching the core and back muscles.

For osteoporosis, incorporate weight-bearing exercises and poses that improve bone density and balance.

Can chair yoga help with cardiovascular health or diabetes management?

Yes, chair yoga can improve cardiovascular health through gentle aerobic activity and reduce stress, which helps manage blood sugar levels in diabetes.

5. How can I modify poses if I have limited mobility or balance issues?

What are some common modifications for traditional yoga poses?

Use a yoga strap to extend your reach.

Place a block under your feet if they don't reach the floor.

Use a cushion for added support on the chair seat.

Are there poses that should be avoided altogether?

Avoid poses that require extreme stretching or bending, or those that cause pain or discomfort. Always prioritize safety and comfort.

6. What breathing techniques are used in chair yoga, and how do they help?

How important is breath control in chair yoga practice?

Breath control is crucial as it helps enhance relaxation, focus, and the effectiveness of the poses.

Can you provide examples of simple breathing exercises?

Diaphragmatic Breathing: Inhale deeply through your nose, expanding your belly, and exhale slowly through your mouth.

Box Breathing: Inhale for a count of 4, hold for 4, exhale for 4, and hold for 4 again. Repeat.

7. How can chair yoga help with mental and emotional well-being?

Are there specific poses or routines that focus on stress relief and relaxation?

Yes, poses like Seated Forward Bend, Seated Cat-Cow, and Gentle Twists help release tension and promote relaxation.

How does mindfulness integrate into chair yoga practice?

Mindfulness is integrated through focused breathing, meditation, and being present in each movement, which helps reduce stress and improve emotional well-being.

8. What resources are available for further learning and practice?

Are there online videos or classes recommended for beginners?

Websites like YouTube have many free chair yoga classes.

Look for instructors specializing in senior yoga.

Online platforms like Yoga with Adriene and the Yoga Journal offer beginner-friendly videos.

What books or articles can provide additional guidance?

Books like "Chair Yoga: Sit, Stretch, and Strengthen Your Way to a Happier, Healthier You" by Kristin McGee are excellent resources.

9. How can I stay motivated and consistent with my practice?

What are some tips for incorporating chair yoga into my daily routine?

Set a regular practice time each day, such as morning or evening.

Use reminders, such as setting alarms or placing your yoga chair and props in a visible spot.

How can I track my progress and set achievable goals?

Keep a yoga journal to record your practice sessions, noting improvements and how you feel.

Set small, achievable goals, like increasing session length gradually or mastering a new pose.

Chapter 3: Understanding Chair Yoga

What is Chair Yoga?
Explanation:
Chair yoga is a gentle form of yoga that adapts traditional yoga poses to be performed while seated or using a chair for support. It allows individuals with physical limitations, seniors, or those recovering from injuries to experience the benefits of yoga in a safe and accessible manner. Chair yoga incorporates modified movements, breath awareness, and mindfulness practices, maintaining the essence of yoga while accommodating diverse needs and abilities.

Addressing Concerns:

Accessibility: Chair yoga is suitable for individuals of all fitness levels and abilities. It eliminates barriers to traditional yoga practices, such as floor-based poses, by offering seated alternatives that promote flexibility, strength, and relaxation.
Effectiveness: Despite being performed from a seated position, chair yoga provides significant physical and mental benefits. It improves flexibility, enhances muscle strength, promotes better posture, and reduces stress levels, making it an effective wellness practice for a wide range of practitioners.
Definition and History
Explanation:

Chair yoga has evolved from traditional yoga practices to meet the needs of modern populations, including seniors and individuals with mobility issues. It originated as a modification of yoga poses to be performed in a seated position or using a chair for stability. The practice has grown in popularity due to its therapeutic benefits and ability to address specific health concerns while maintaining the foundational principles of yoga.

Addressing Concerns:

Authenticity: Chair yoga retains core aspects of traditional yoga, such as breath control (pranayama), mindfulness, and alignment principles. It adapts these elements to suit seated postures and movements, ensuring authenticity while enhancing accessibility.
Development: Over time, chair yoga has adapted to include a variety of poses and techniques that cater to diverse health conditions and lifestyles. Its evolution reflects ongoing research and innovation in yoga therapy, making it a valuable practice for promoting overall well-being.
Differences between Traditional Yoga and Chair Yoga
Explanation:
The primary difference between traditional yoga and chair yoga lies in the adaptation of poses and practices to accommodate physical limitations and accessibility challenges. Traditional yoga often involves dynamic movements, standing poses, and floor-based exercises that require strength and flexibility. In contrast, chair yoga focuses on seated poses, gentle stretches, and modified movements that utilize a chair for support.

Addressing Concerns:

Benefits Comparison: Chair yoga offers similar benefits to traditional yoga, such as improved flexibility, strength, and relaxation, albeit from a seated position. It provides stability and support, making it suitable for seniors, individuals with balance issues, or those recovering from injury.

Safety Considerations: Chair yoga minimizes the risk of strain or injury associated with more demanding yoga practices. It emphasizes proper alignment, gradual progression, and adaptations tailored to individual needs, ensuring a safe and effective exercise option for diverse populations.

Benefits of Chair Yoga

Physical Benefits:

Improved Flexibility: Chair yoga incorporates gentle stretches and movements that help maintain and enhance joint flexibility and range of motion. These exercises reduce stiffness and promote suppleness in muscles and connective tissues.

Enhanced Strength: Seated poses and resistance exercises in chair yoga strengthen muscles, particularly in the core, arms, and legs. This improves overall stability, posture, and functional strength.

Better Balance: Balance-focused exercises in a seated position enhance proprioception and stability, reducing the risk of falls and increasing confidence in movement.

Mental Benefits:

Stress Reduction: Chair yoga integrates breath-centered practices and relaxation techniques that activate the parasympathetic nervous system. This promotes deep relaxation, reduces stress levels, and supports emotional well-being.

Mental Clarity: Mindfulness exercises in chair yoga enhance focus, concentration, and cognitive function. They cultivate present-moment awareness, which fosters mental clarity, resilience, and a positive mindset.

Emotional Well-being: Engaging in chair yoga fosters a sense of calm, inner peace, and emotional balance. It encourages self-awareness, emotional resilience, and a deeper connection between mind and body.

Chapter Outline

Breathing Techniques

Explanation:

Breath awareness (pranayama) is integral to chair yoga practice, serving as a foundation for linking breath with movement and promoting relaxation. Chair yoga includes simple breathing exercises that enhance oxygenation, calm the mind, and facilitate a mindful state during practice.

Addressing Concerns:

Accessibility: Breathing exercises in chair yoga are accessible to individuals of all ages and fitness levels. They can be adapted to accommodate respiratory conditions or varying breathing capacities, ensuring comfort and effectiveness.

Benefits: Breathing techniques in chair yoga immediately alleviate stress, improve focus, and enhance overall relaxation response. They provide a practical tool for managing daily stressors and promoting mental clarity.

Basic Postures

Explanation:

Chair yoga offers a range of seated poses that promote flexibility, strength, and relaxation. These include foundational poses such as Seated Mountain Pose, Seated Twist, and Seated Forward Fold, which are adapted to be comfortably performed with the support of a chair.

Addressing Concerns:

Adaptability: Chair yoga poses can be modified to accommodate individual needs and limitations. Variations using props like yoga straps or blocks help practitioners adjust poses for comfort and safety, encouraging gradual progression and improvement.

Safety Guidelines: Provide clear instructions on proper alignment, breathing techniques, and modifications for each pose. Emphasize the importance of practicing within one's limits to prevent strain or injury, promoting a sustainable and enjoyable yoga experience.

Warm-up Exercises

Explanation:

Warm-up exercises are essential in chair yoga to prepare the body for movement, increase circulation, and prevent injury. These gentle exercises include neck stretches, shoulder rolls, and seated twists that promote joint mobility and enhance flexibility.

Addressing Concerns:

Importance of Warm-up: Emphasize the role of warm-up exercises in chair yoga to optimize physical readiness and improve the effectiveness of subsequent poses. Warm-ups reduce muscle tension, increase blood flow to tissues, and enhance overall comfort during practice.

Integration into Routine: Encourage readers to incorporate warm-up exercises into their chair yoga routine as a foundational step. Provide a sequence of warm-up movements that can be easily performed at home or in a class setting, fostering consistency and progress in practice.

Examples of Warm-Up Exercises for Chair Yoga

Neck Stretches:

Neck Rolls: Sit comfortably in a chair with feet flat on the floor. Slowly drop your chin towards your chest and roll your head gently from side to side in a half-circle motion. Repeat 5-10 times.
Neck Tilts: Sit tall and gently tilt your head to one side, bringing your ear towards your shoulder. Hold for a few breaths, then switch sides. Repeat 3-5 times on each side.
Shoulder Rolls:

Shoulder Circles: Sit tall with arms relaxed by your sides. Inhale as you lift your shoulders towards your ears, exhale as you roll them back and down. Repeat 5-10 times, then reverse the direction.
Shoulder Shrugs: Lift both shoulders towards your ears as you inhale deeply, hold briefly, then exhale as you release them down. Repeat 5-10 times to release tension in the shoulders.
Seated Twists:

Spinal Twist: Sit up tall with feet flat on the floor. Inhale to lengthen the spine, then exhale as you twist gently to the right, placing your left hand on the outside of your right knee and your right hand on the back of the chair. Hold for a few breaths, then switch sides. Repeat 3-5 times on each side.
Arm and Wrist Stretches:

Wrist Circles: Extend your arms in front of you with palms facing down. Make gentle circles with your wrists in one direction, then reverse. Repeat 5-10 times each direction to increase circulation and flexibility in the wrists and forearms.
Arm Extensions: Extend one arm overhead, palm facing inward. Reach up and over to the opposite side, feeling a stretch along the side of your body. Hold for a few breaths, then switch sides. Repeat 3-5 times on each side.
Hip and Leg Movements:

Seated Leg Extensions: Sit with feet flat on the floor. Extend one leg forward, heel on the floor, toes pointing up. Hold for a few breaths, then switch legs. Repeat 3-5 times on each leg to stretch the hamstrings and calf muscles.
Ankle Circles: Lift one foot off the floor and make gentle circles with your ankle in one direction, then reverse. Repeat 5-10 times each direction to improve ankle mobility and circulation.
Deep Breathing Exercises:

Diaphragmatic Breathing: Sit tall with hands on your belly. Inhale deeply through your nose, allowing your belly to expand with air. Exhale slowly through your mouth, drawing your belly button towards your spine. Repeat for several cycles to calm the nervous system and prepare for relaxation.
Tips for Incorporating Warm-Up Exercises:
Begin with gentle movements and gradually increase intensity as your body warms up.

Focus on smooth, controlled movements and synchronize your breath with each exercise.
Pay attention to any areas of tension or discomfort, modifying exercises as needed to suit your body's needs.
Use props like a chair, yoga strap, or cushion for support and stability during stretches and movements.
These warm-up exercises help prepare the body for chair yoga practice by increasing circulation, enhancing flexibility, and reducing muscle tension. Incorporate them into your routine to optimize the benefits of chair yoga and promote overall well-being.

Chapter 4: What is Chair Yoga?

Chair yoga is a modified form of yoga that adapts traditional yoga poses and principles to be performed while seated or with the support of a chair. This chapter explores the essence of chair yoga, its techniques, and the myriad benefits it offers to practitioners of all ages and abilities.

Exploring Chair Yoga
Introduction to Chair Yoga:
Chair yoga is introduced as a gentle and accessible form of yoga suitable for individuals with mobility issues, seniors, office workers, and anyone looking to enjoy the benefits of yoga without the need for complex movements or standing poses. It highlights how chair yoga combines the wisdom of traditional yoga with modifications that make it safe and effective for diverse populations.

Core Principles of Chair Yoga
Adaptation of Traditional Poses:

Chair yoga adapts classic yoga postures to be performed while seated on a chair or using a chair for support. It emphasizes modifications that cater to individuals with limited mobility, joint stiffness, or balance concerns. This section outlines how each pose is adjusted to maintain its essence while ensuring comfort and safety.

Breath Awareness and Mindfulness:
Similar to traditional yoga, chair yoga incorporates breath awareness (pranayama) and mindfulness techniques. It emphasizes the synchronization of breath with movement, promoting relaxation, reducing stress levels, and enhancing mental clarity. Techniques such as deep belly breathing and alternate nostril breathing are explained in detail.

Benefits of Chair Yoga
Physical Benefits:
Chair yoga promotes physical well-being by improving flexibility, strength, and balance. It includes gentle stretches and movements that target major muscle groups while reducing stiffness and enhancing joint mobility. Specific benefits for seniors, such as maintaining bone density and improving posture, are highlighted.

Mental and Emotional Well-being:
The practice of chair yoga supports mental health by reducing anxiety, improving mood, and increasing resilience to stress. Mindfulness exercises foster a sense of inner peace and emotional stability. This section discusses how chair yoga can enhance cognitive function and promote a positive outlook on life.

Techniques and Practices
Seated Postures and Sequences:

Detailed instructions are provided for foundational chair yoga poses and sequences. This includes poses like Seated Mountain Pose, Seated Forward Fold, and Gentle Twist, along with variations and modifications. Each pose is accompanied by guidance on alignment, breathing techniques, and the benefits it offers.

Warm-up and Cool-down Routines:
Effective warm-up exercises are essential to prepare the body for chair yoga practice, promoting circulation and flexibility. Cool-down sequences help to relax muscles and restore calmness after a session. Sample routines and their benefits are outlined to encourage a balanced practice.

Advanced Chair Yoga Practices
Progression and Challenges:
For those looking to deepen their practice, advanced chair yoga poses and sequences are introduced. These include poses that incorporate more challenging movements, such as balancing exercises and strength-building postures. Safety tips and gradual progression guidelines are emphasized.

Specialized Applications
Chair Yoga for Specific Health Conditions:
Tailored chair yoga routines are provided for managing common health concerns such as arthritis, back pain, cardiovascular health, osteoporosis, and diabetes. Each routine includes poses and practices designed to alleviate symptoms and promote overall well-being.

Integration into Daily Life
Incorporating Chair Yoga Off the Mat:
Practical tips are offered for integrating chair yoga into daily routines, whether at home, in the office, or while traveling. Strategies for maintaining consistency in practice and overcoming barriers to regular exercise are discussed.

Conclusion
Recap of Benefits and Encouragement:
The chapter concludes with a summary of the benefits of chair
yoga, reinforcing its accessibility and positive impact on
physical, mental, and emotional health. Readers are
encouraged to explore chair yoga as a sustainable and
enjoyable wellness practice.

By exploring these aspects comprehensively, Chapter 4 on
Chair Yoga provides readers with a thorough understanding
of what chair yoga entails, its benefits, and practical
techniques to incorporate into their daily lives. It serves as a
guide to empower individuals of all ages and abilities to
embark on a journey of health and well-being through chair
yoga.
Practical Application:

Finding a Chair Yoga Class:
Finding a chair yoga class near you involves exploring local
resources:

Community Centers or Gyms: These often host chair yoga
classes tailored for various age groups, including seniors.
Check their schedules or websites for class times and
availability.
Senior Centers: Many senior centers offer chair yoga sessions
as part of their wellness programs. Contact them directly or
check community bulletin boards for information.
Online Directories: Websites like YogaFinder, Mindbody, or
local community event listings can help locate nearby classes.
Instructor Referrals: If you attend other yoga classes, ask
instructors if they offer chair yoga or can recommend classes
in your area.
Practicing Chair Yoga at Home:

Environment Setup: Choose a quiet, clutter-free space where you can place a sturdy chair with a flat seat and backrest. Ensure there's ample room around you to stretch comfortably.
Props and Equipment: Gather essential props such as yoga blocks, straps, or blankets to modify poses and provide support as needed.
Online Resources: Utilize online platforms offering guided chair yoga videos or written routines. Look for reputable sources that provide clear instructions and adaptations for beginners.
Choosing the Right Chair:

Ideal Chair Characteristics: Select a chair with a firm seat and backrest that supports your spine comfortably. Avoid chairs with wheels or armrests that restrict movement.
Safety Considerations: Ensure the chair's height allows your feet to rest flat on the floor, promoting stability during poses. Modify poses by using cushions or folded blankets for added support and comfort.
Health and Safety Concerns:

Precautions for Health Conditions:

Consultation with Healthcare Provider: Before starting chair yoga, consult your healthcare provider, especially if you have pre-existing health conditions or injuries. Discuss any limitations or concerns to receive personalized guidance on safe practice.
Modifications and Alternatives: Your healthcare provider can recommend specific modifications or alternative poses that accommodate your health needs, ensuring you practice safely and effectively.
Correct Pose Alignment:

Guidance from Qualified Instructors: Attend classes led by certified chair yoga instructors who offer individualized attention and guidance on proper pose alignment.

Body Awareness: Listen to your body's signals during practice. Avoid pushing into discomfort or pain, and use props like blocks or straps to maintain correct alignment and support.

Safety for Seniors:

Gradual Progression: Start with gentle poses and gradually increase intensity as you become more comfortable and confident.

Balance and Stability: Chair yoga promotes balance through seated poses and stability exercises, reducing the risk of falls and enhancing confidence in movement.

Effectiveness and Benefits:

Improvements in Flexibility and Strength:

Consistent Practice: Regular chair yoga practice, even a few times per week, can enhance flexibility and muscle strength noticeably over time.

Focus on Range of Motion: Chair yoga emphasizes gentle stretches that increase joint mobility and improve flexibility throughout the body.

Specific Health Benefits:

Arthritis or Joint Pain: Chair yoga routines include gentle movements that alleviate stiffness and enhance joint flexibility, making it beneficial for managing symptoms of arthritis.

Back Pain: Strengthening exercises and gentle stretches in chair yoga help relieve tension in the back muscles and promote better spinal alignment.

Mental Benefits:

Stress Reduction: Breath-centered practices and relaxation techniques in chair yoga activate the body's relaxation response, reducing stress levels and promoting a sense of calm.

Cognitive Function: Mindfulness exercises improve focus, concentration, and mental clarity, supporting overall cognitive function and emotional well-being.

Progression and Challenges:

Advancing in Chair Yoga:

Gradual Challenges: As you become more proficient, explore advanced chair yoga poses that incorporate balance, strength, and flexibility.

Instructor Guidance: Seek guidance from experienced instructors who can suggest modifications or variations to suit your evolving practice level and prevent plateaus.

Common Challenges and Solutions:

Physical Limitations: Modify poses to suit your abilities, focusing on gradual progression and using props for support as needed.

Consistency: Establish a regular chair yoga practice routine to experience ongoing benefits. Set achievable goals and track progress to stay motivated.

Integration into Daily Life:

Practice Frequency:

Recommended Frequency: Aim for consistency with chair yoga practice, ideally 2-3 sessions per week to maintain and build upon benefits like flexibility, strength, and stress reduction.

Short Sessions: Incorporate brief chair yoga routines during breaks at work or between daily activities to refresh and rejuvenate your body and mind.

Complementing Other Practices:

Synergy with Other Activities: Chair yoga can complement activities such as walking, swimming, or other forms of exercise, enhancing overall fitness and flexibility.
Holistic Approach: Combine chair yoga with mindfulness practices or relaxation techniques for a comprehensive approach to well-being and stress management.
Community and Resources:

Online Resources:

Guided Videos and Classes: Access reputable online platforms offering guided chair yoga videos or live-streamed classes that you can participate in from the comfort of your home.
Community Forums: Engage with online communities or forums dedicated to chair yoga, where you can connect with others, share experiences, ask questions, and find support.
Recommended Reading and Further Study:

Books and Articles: Explore recommended reading materials authored by experts in yoga therapy and senior fitness, offering deeper insights into chair yoga techniques, benefits, and applications.
Continuing Education: Consider attending workshops, seminars, or advanced chair yoga classes to expand your knowledge and refine your practice under expert guidance.

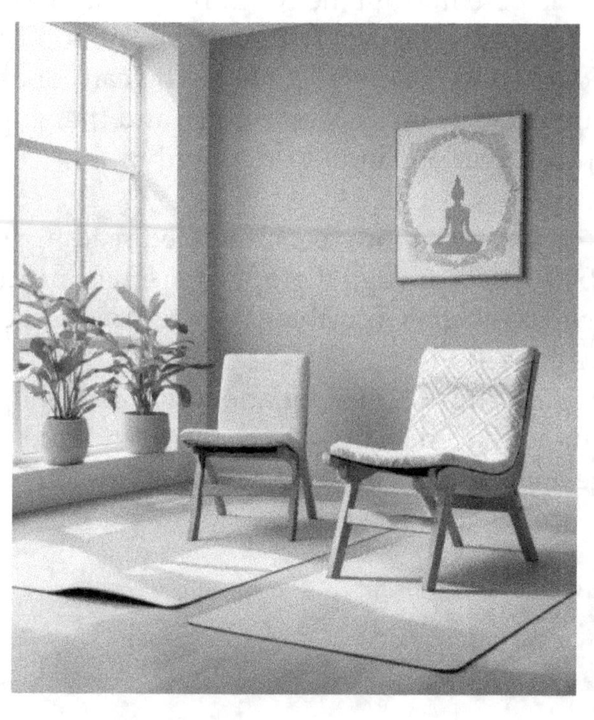

Chapter 5: Understanding Chair Yoga

Definition and History
Definition of Chair Yoga:
Chair yoga is a gentle form of yoga that can be practiced while seated in a chair or standing using a chair for support. This adaptation makes yoga accessible to individuals who may have mobility issues, balance concerns, or difficulty practicing traditional yoga on the floor. Chair yoga includes modifications of traditional yoga poses, breathing exercises, and relaxation techniques, all tailored to be performed comfortably while sitting or using a chair for balance.

Key Elements of Chair Yoga:

Seated Poses: Adaptations of traditional yoga postures that can be performed while sitting in a chair.

Standing Poses: Yoga poses performed while using a chair for support and balance.

Breathing Exercises: Techniques to promote relaxation and enhance respiratory function.

Mindfulness and Relaxation: Practices aimed at reducing stress and promoting mental clarity.

History of Chair Yoga:

Chair yoga emerged as a specialized practice in the latter half of the 20th century, designed to make yoga accessible to everyone, regardless of physical limitations. Its development is linked to the broader movement of adaptive yoga, which aims to modify traditional yoga practices to meet the needs of diverse populations.

Origins and Evolution:

Early Development: The concept of modifying yoga for those with limited mobility has roots in the early days of yoga's introduction to the West. Teachers began to recognize the need for adaptations to make yoga more inclusive.

Key Figures: Various yoga instructors and therapists have contributed to the development and popularization of chair yoga. Notable among them is Lakshmi Voelker, who is often credited with formalizing chair yoga in the 1980s. Voelker created a structured program called "Chair Yoga" to serve her clients who had difficulty practicing traditional yoga.

Growth and Popularity: Chair yoga has grown significantly over the past few decades, with classes now offered in community centers, senior living facilities, rehabilitation centers, and online platforms. The practice is recognized for its ability to improve flexibility, strength, balance, and mental well-being without the need for getting on the floor.

Cultural Context and Adaptation:

Chair yoga's evolution has been influenced by the broader acceptance and integration of yoga into Western culture. Its adaptation addresses the specific needs of populations such as seniors, individuals with disabilities, and those recovering from injuries, making the benefits of yoga accessible to a wider audience.

Current Practice:
Today, chair yoga is widely practiced and respected for its therapeutic benefits. It is used in various settings, including:

Senior Centers and Assisted Living Facilities: Offering seniors a way to stay active and engaged.
Rehabilitation Clinics: Assisting individuals recovering from surgery or injury.
Workplaces: Providing a break from sedentary work environments to improve overall wellness.
Online Platforms: Making chair yoga accessible to people at home through videos and live-streamed classes.
Benefits of Chair Yoga:

Physical Benefits: Improves flexibility, muscle strength, and balance while reducing the risk of injury.
Mental Benefits: Enhances mental clarity, reduces stress, and promotes relaxation.
Emotional and Social Benefits: Provides a sense of community, reduces feelings of isolation, and boosts overall emotional well-being.
Understanding the definition and history of chair yoga helps appreciate its significance and the thoughtful adaptations that make yoga accessible to everyone, regardless of physical ability. Chair yoga stands as a testament to yoga's adaptability and the commitment to inclusivity within the yoga community.

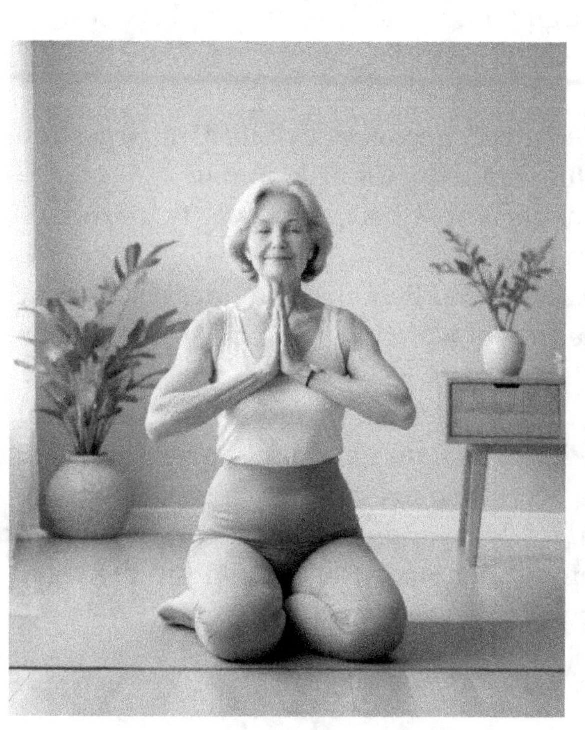

Chapter 6: Differences Between Traditional Yoga and Chair Yoga

Introduction:
While traditional yoga and chair yoga share the same foundational principles, such as breath control, mindfulness, and physical postures, they differ significantly in their approach, execution, and target audience. Understanding these differences can help individuals choose the best practice for their needs and abilities.

Key Differences
Accessibility and Inclusivity:

Traditional Yoga: Often requires a certain level of physical fitness and mobility, making it less accessible to individuals with limited movement, seniors, or those with specific health conditions.

Chair Yoga: Designed to be inclusive and accessible to everyone, regardless of age, fitness level, or physical ability. It removes barriers by allowing participants to practice yoga while seated or using a chair for support.

Physical Demands and Postures:

Traditional Yoga: Involves a wide range of poses, including standing, balancing, sitting, and lying down on a mat. Poses often require significant flexibility, strength, and balance.

Chair Yoga: Adapts traditional poses to be performed while seated or using a chair for support. This reduces the physical demands, making it suitable for those with limited strength, flexibility, or balance. Poses are modified to ensure they can be performed comfortably and safely.

Balance and Stability:

Traditional Yoga: Many poses, especially balancing poses, require the ability to maintain stability on one leg or in a challenging position, which can be difficult for those with balance issues.

Chair Yoga: Emphasizes stability and safety by providing the chair as a constant support, reducing the risk of falls or loss of balance. This focus on stability makes it ideal for older adults and those with balance concerns.

Intensity and Pace:

Traditional Yoga: Can range from gentle to vigorous, with styles like Vinyasa or Ashtanga involving dynamic sequences and rapid transitions between poses.

Chair Yoga: Generally focuses on gentle, slow-paced movements that prioritize safety and comfort. It emphasizes mindful movement and controlled breathing, making it ideal for relaxation and stress relief.
Breathing Techniques:

Traditional Yoga: While breath control (pranayama) is integral, it can be challenging to maintain proper breathing techniques during complex or strenuous poses.
Chair Yoga: Places a strong emphasis on breathing exercises that can be easily performed while seated. This focus helps enhance respiratory function and promotes relaxation.
Adaptations and Modifications:

Traditional Yoga: Modifications are often available for beginners or those with specific limitations, but the need for a full range of motion can still be a barrier.
Chair Yoga: Entirely based on adaptations, it offers numerous modifications for each pose to accommodate various physical limitations. This ensures that every participant can practice safely and effectively.
Target Audience:

Traditional Yoga: Attracts a broad audience, including fitness enthusiasts, athletes, and individuals seeking a comprehensive physical workout.
Chair Yoga: Specifically targets seniors, individuals with disabilities, those recovering from injuries, and anyone seeking a gentle, supportive yoga practice.
Benefits Specific to Chair Yoga
Enhanced Accessibility: Provides a way for those who may not be able to participate in traditional yoga to still enjoy the benefits of yoga.
Improved Joint Health: Gentle movements promote joint flexibility without putting stress on the joints.

Mental and Emotional Well-being: Promotes relaxation, reduces stress, and can be practiced in a supportive group environment, enhancing social interaction.
Functional Fitness: Focuses on movements that improve daily functioning, such as reaching, bending, and standing up from a seated position.
Examples of Pose Adaptations
Seated Forward Bend (Paschimottanasana):

Traditional Yoga: Performed sitting on the floor with legs extended, bending forward to touch the toes.
Chair Yoga: Performed sitting in a chair, extending the legs slightly forward, and bending at the waist to reach toward the feet.
Warrior Pose (Virabhadrasana):

Traditional Yoga: Involves standing with legs apart, bending one knee, and extending the arms overhead or to the sides.
Chair Yoga: Can be performed sitting with one leg bent at the knee and the other extended to the side, arms raised to shoulder height.
Tree Pose (Vrksasana):

Traditional Yoga: Balancing on one leg with the other foot placed on the inner thigh or calf, hands in prayer position.
Chair Yoga: Performed standing with one hand on the chair for support, placing the other foot on the ankle or calf, and raising one arm.
Conclusion

Understanding the differences between traditional yoga and chair yoga highlights the adaptability and inclusiveness of chair yoga. By modifying traditional poses and focusing on safety and accessibility, chair yoga provides a valuable opportunity for individuals of all abilities to enjoy the physical, mental, and emotional benefits of yoga. This gentle practice ensures that yoga's transformative potential is available to everyone, promoting a healthier, more active, and balanced lifestyle.

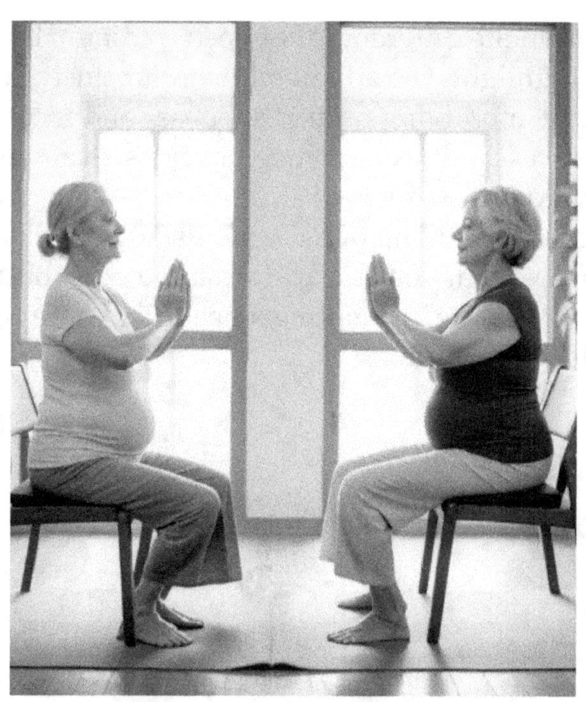

Chapter 7: Benefits of Chair Yoga

Chair yoga offers a wide range of benefits that cater to the physical, mental, emotional, and social well-being of individuals, particularly seniors and those with limited mobility. This chapter will delve into these benefits, providing a comprehensive understanding of how chair yoga can enhance overall health and quality of life.

Physical Benefits
Improved Flexibility:

Gentle Stretching: Chair yoga involves gentle stretches that help increase the flexibility of muscles and joints, enhancing the range of motion and reducing stiffness.
Joint Mobility: Regular practice can help maintain and even improve joint mobility, crucial for daily activities.
Increased Strength:

Muscle Engagement: Chair yoga poses are designed to engage various muscle groups, building strength without the need for intense physical effort.
Core Stability: Strengthening the core muscles can improve overall stability and support better posture.
Better Balance:

Safe Environment: Using a chair for support, individuals can practice balance poses safely, reducing the risk of falls.
Coordination: Chair yoga helps improve coordination, an essential factor for preventing falls and enhancing overall mobility.
Enhanced Circulation:

Movement: Gentle movements in chair yoga promote better blood circulation, helping to deliver oxygen and nutrients throughout the body.
Breathing Exercises: Controlled breathing can also enhance circulation and improve cardiovascular health.
Pain Management:

Reduced Joint Pain: Chair yoga can help alleviate symptoms of arthritis and other joint conditions by promoting gentle movement and flexibility.
Back Pain Relief: Specific poses target back muscles, providing relief from chronic back pain and improving spinal health.
Mental Benefits
Stress Reduction:

Relaxation Techniques: Chair yoga incorporates relaxation techniques that help reduce stress levels and promote a sense of calm.
Mindfulness: Practicing mindfulness during yoga helps individuals stay present, reducing anxiety and stress.
Improved Mental Clarity:

Focus and Concentration: The mindful practice of chair yoga enhances focus and concentration, which can improve cognitive function.
Mental Calmness: Regular practice can lead to a quieter mind, reducing mental clutter and enhancing clarity.
Enhanced Mood:

Endorphin Release: Physical activity and mindful breathing stimulate the release of endorphins, the body's natural mood lifters.
Positive Outlook: The sense of achievement and well-being gained from regular practice can improve overall mood and outlook on life.
Emotional and Social Benefits

Emotional Well-being:

Stress Relief: Reducing stress through chair yoga can lead to better emotional regulation and reduced feelings of anxiety and depression.
Self-Confidence: Successfully engaging in chair yoga can boost self-esteem and confidence, especially for those who may feel limited by their physical abilities.
Social Interaction:

Group Classes: Participating in chair yoga classes provides an opportunity for social interaction, fostering a sense of community and belonging.
Support Networks: Building connections with fellow practitioners can create a support network, reducing feelings of isolation.
Enhanced Quality of Life:

Daily Functioning: The physical and mental benefits of chair yoga translate into better performance of daily activities, enhancing independence and quality of life.
Holistic Well-being: The comprehensive benefits of chair yoga contribute to an overall sense of well-being, balancing physical health with mental and emotional stability.
Specific Benefits for Health Conditions
Arthritis and Joint Pain:

Gentle Movement: Chair yoga provides gentle movement that can reduce joint pain and stiffness associated with arthritis.
Inflammation Reduction: Regular practice may help reduce inflammation in the joints, improving overall joint health.
Back Pain:

Strengthening Exercises: Chair yoga poses that strengthen the back and core muscles can alleviate chronic back pain.

Postural Alignment: Improved posture from chair yoga can help prevent and relieve back pain.
Cardiovascular Health:

Heart-Healthy Poses: Specific poses and breathing exercises in chair yoga can support heart health by improving circulation and reducing stress.
Blood Pressure Management: The stress-reducing effects of chair yoga can help manage blood pressure levels.
Osteoporosis:

Bone Density: Weight-bearing poses in chair yoga can help maintain and improve bone density, crucial for individuals with osteoporosis.
Fall Prevention: Improved balance and strength reduce the risk of falls, which is particularly important for those with fragile bones.
Diabetes:

Blood Sugar Control: Regular physical activity, including chair yoga, helps manage blood sugar levels, supporting diabetes management.
Improved Circulation: Enhanced circulation from yoga practice can aid in preventing complications related to diabetes.
Conclusion
Chair yoga offers a wide array of benefits that cater to the physical, mental, emotional, and social needs of practitioners. Its gentle, accessible approach makes it particularly suitable for seniors and those with limited mobility, ensuring that everyone can enjoy the transformative effects of yoga. By incorporating chair yoga into your routine, you can experience improved flexibility, strength, balance, mental clarity, and overall well-being, leading to a healthier, more active, and fulfilling life.

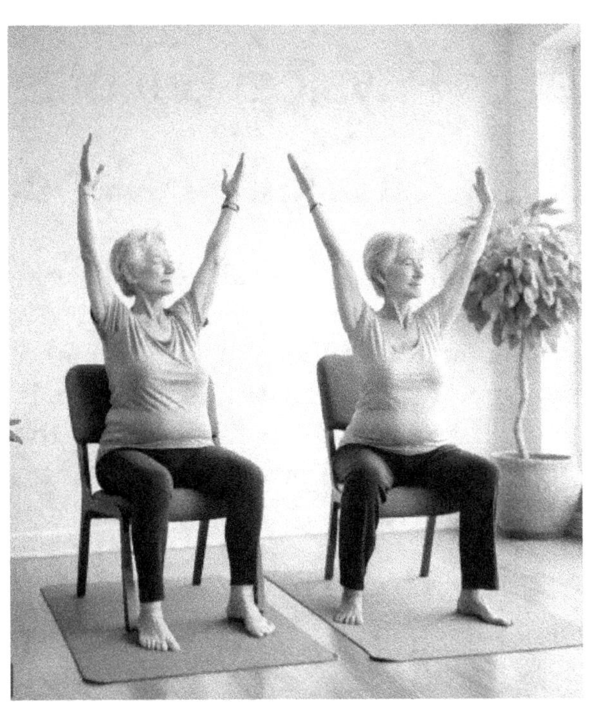

Chapter 8: Physical Benefits (Flexibility, Strength, Balance)

Chair yoga offers numerous physical benefits, particularly in enhancing flexibility, strength, and balance. These benefits are crucial for maintaining overall health, independence, and quality of life, especially for seniors and individuals with limited mobility. In this chapter, we will explore these physical benefits in detail and provide insights into how chair yoga can help improve them.

Flexibility
Improved Range of Motion:

Gentle Stretching: Chair yoga involves gentle stretching exercises that target various muscle groups and joints. These stretches help increase the range of motion, making everyday activities easier and more comfortable.
Joint Health: Regular stretching keeps the joints lubricated and flexible, reducing the risk of stiffness and discomfort. This is particularly beneficial for individuals with arthritis or other joint-related issues.
Muscle Flexibility:

Targeted Stretches: Chair yoga poses are designed to stretch specific muscles, improving their elasticity and reducing the risk of injury. For example, seated forward bends stretch the hamstrings and lower back, while seated twists enhance spinal flexibility.
Consistency: Practicing chair yoga regularly helps maintain and gradually improve muscle flexibility, contributing to overall physical health.
Strength

Building Muscle Strength:

Resistance and Weight-Bearing: Chair yoga incorporates poses that use body weight and resistance to build muscle strength. Even without intense physical exertion, these poses effectively engage and strengthen various muscle groups.
Core Stability: Strengthening the core muscles, including the abdomen and lower back, is a key focus in chair yoga. A strong core enhances overall stability and supports better posture.
Functional Strength:

Daily Activities: The strength gained from chair yoga translates into improved performance of daily activities, such as lifting objects, standing up from a seated position, and walking. This functional strength is essential for maintaining independence.
Preventing Muscle Loss: As we age, maintaining muscle mass becomes increasingly important. Chair yoga helps counteract age-related muscle loss by providing a gentle yet effective form of strength training.
Balance
Enhanced Stability:

Balance Poses: Chair yoga includes balance poses that are performed with the support of a chair. These poses help improve overall stability and coordination, reducing the risk of falls and injuries.
Proprioception: Practicing balance poses enhances proprioception, which is the body's ability to sense its position and movement in space. Improved proprioception leads to better balance and coordination.
Fall Prevention:

Safe Practice Environment: By providing a safe and supportive environment, chair yoga allows individuals to practice balance exercises without the fear of falling. This builds confidence and encourages continued practice.
Strength and Flexibility Integration: The combination of increased strength and flexibility from chair yoga contributes to better balance. Strong muscles and flexible joints work together to maintain stability and prevent falls.
Specific Chair Yoga Exercises for Physical Benefits
Flexibility Exercises:

Seated Forward Bend: Sit with your legs extended and gently reach forward towards your feet. This stretches the hamstrings and lower back.
Seated Side Stretch: Sit upright and reach one arm overhead, gently bending to the opposite side. This stretches the sides of the torso and improves spinal flexibility.
Strength Exercises:

Seated Leg Lifts: Sit with your back straight and lift one leg at a time, keeping it extended. This strengthens the quadriceps and hip flexors.
Chair Push-Ups: Place your hands on the arms of the chair and push yourself up slightly, engaging the upper body muscles, particularly the triceps and shoulders.
Balance Exercises:

Chair-Assisted Tree Pose: Stand beside the chair, holding it for support. Place one foot on the opposite ankle or calf, balancing on the standing leg. This improves balance and stability.
Seated Marching: Sit upright and march in place, lifting each knee towards the chest. This enhances coordination and balance.
Conclusion

Chair yoga provides a safe, effective way to improve flexibility, strength, and balance. These physical benefits are essential for maintaining overall health, independence, and quality of life, especially for seniors and those with limited mobility. By incorporating chair yoga into your routine, you can enhance your physical capabilities and enjoy a more active and fulfilling lifestyle.

Chapter 9: Mental Benefits (Stress Reduction, Mental Clarity)

Chair yoga is not only beneficial for physical health but also significantly enhances mental well-being. This chapter explores how chair yoga can help reduce stress and improve mental clarity, contributing to a balanced and peaceful mind.

Stress Reduction
Relaxation Techniques:

Breathing Exercises: Chair yoga incorporates deep, mindful breathing exercises that activate the parasympathetic nervous system, promoting relaxation and reducing the body's stress response. Techniques such as diaphragmatic breathing and alternate nostril breathing can calm the mind and lower stress levels.
Progressive Muscle Relaxation: This technique involves tensing and then slowly releasing different muscle groups, which can help alleviate physical tension associated with stress.
Mindfulness and Meditation:

Present Moment Awareness: Chair yoga emphasizes mindfulness, encouraging practitioners to focus on the present moment. This can help reduce anxiety and prevent the mind from wandering to stressful thoughts about the past or future.
Guided Meditation: Integrating guided meditation sessions into chair yoga practice can enhance relaxation and provide a mental break from stressors.
Physical Movement:

Gentle Movement: Engaging in gentle, rhythmic movements can help release endorphins, the body's natural stress relievers. Movements such as seated cat-cow stretches or gentle twists can reduce tension and promote a sense of well-being.

Release of Muscle Tension: Chair yoga helps release physical tension held in the muscles, which can be a physical manifestation of stress. By easing this tension, mental stress is also alleviated.

Mental Clarity

Enhanced Focus and Concentration:

Concentration on Breath: The practice of focusing on breath during chair yoga sessions improves concentration and trains the mind to stay present. This enhanced focus can carry over into daily activities, improving overall cognitive function.

Mental Discipline: Regular practice of chair yoga helps develop mental discipline, making it easier to concentrate on tasks and reduce distractions.

Cognitive Function:

Neuroplasticity: Engaging in chair yoga can stimulate brain function and promote neuroplasticity, the brain's ability to reorganize itself by forming new neural connections. This can improve memory, learning, and other cognitive functions.

Mind-Body Connection: Strengthening the mind-body connection through chair yoga can enhance mental clarity and awareness, making it easier to navigate complex thoughts and tasks.

Emotional Regulation:

Balanced Emotions: Chair yoga promotes emotional balance by regulating the body's stress hormones, such as cortisol. Lower stress levels contribute to a more stable mood and improved emotional health.

Positive Outlook: Regular practice of chair yoga can lead to a more positive outlook on life. The sense of accomplishment from practicing yoga and the physical release of endorphins can enhance overall mood and mental well-being.
Examples of Chair Yoga Practices for Mental Benefits:

Stress Reduction:

Seated Forward Bend: This pose can help calm the mind and relieve stress. Sit on the chair with feet flat on the floor, extend your arms forward, and gently bend at the hips, reaching towards your toes. Hold the pose for several breaths, focusing on slow, deep breathing.
Alternate Nostril Breathing: This breathing technique can balance the nervous system and reduce stress. Sit comfortably, use your right thumb to close your right nostril, inhale deeply through the left nostril, then close the left nostril with your ring finger and exhale through the right nostril. Continue alternating for several breaths.
Mental Clarity:

Seated Twist: This pose improves spinal flexibility and stimulates the digestive system, which can enhance mental clarity. Sit upright with feet flat on the floor, twist your torso to the right, placing your left hand on your right knee and your right hand on the chair back. Hold for several breaths, then switch sides.
Mindfulness Meditation: End your chair yoga session with a few minutes of mindfulness meditation. Sit comfortably with your eyes closed, focus on your breath, and let go of any thoughts that arise. This practice can clear the mind and improve focus.
Conclusion

Chair yoga offers substantial mental benefits, including stress reduction and improved mental clarity. Through mindful breathing, gentle movements, and meditation, chair yoga helps calm the mind, enhance focus, and promote emotional balance. These mental benefits contribute to a healthier, more relaxed, and clearer state of mind, enhancing overall quality of life. Incorporating chair yoga into your routine can lead to lasting improvements in mental well-being, making it a valuable practice for individuals of all ages and abilities.

Chapter 10: Emotional and Social Benefits

Chair yoga extends beyond physical and mental improvements to provide significant emotional and social benefits. These aspects are crucial for holistic well-being, particularly for seniors and individuals with limited mobility. This chapter will explore how chair yoga enhances emotional health and fosters social connections, contributing to a more fulfilling and balanced life.

Emotional Benefits
Stress Relief and Emotional Regulation:

Calming Effects: Chair yoga incorporates deep breathing and relaxation techniques that activate the parasympathetic nervous system, promoting a state of calm and reducing emotional stress.
Emotional Stability: Regular practice can help regulate the body's stress hormones, such as cortisol, leading to more balanced emotions and improved emotional health.
Increased Self-Esteem and Confidence:

Sense of Accomplishment: Successfully performing chair yoga poses and routines can boost self-esteem and confidence, especially for those who may feel limited by their physical abilities.
Positive Body Image: Engaging in chair yoga promotes a positive relationship with one's body, enhancing body image and self-acceptance.
Emotional Release and Healing:

Releasing Tension: Chair yoga helps release physical tension stored in the body, which can be linked to emotional stress. This release can lead to emotional healing and a sense of relief.
Mind-Body Connection: By fostering a strong mind-body connection, chair yoga encourages emotional awareness and expression, facilitating emotional healing and growth.
Enhanced Mood and Happiness:

Endorphin Release: Physical activity, including chair yoga, stimulates the release of endorphins, the body's natural mood enhancers. This can lead to improved mood and a greater sense of happiness.
Mindfulness and Gratitude: Practicing mindfulness during chair yoga encourages a focus on the present moment and fosters a sense of gratitude, contributing to overall emotional well-being.
Social Benefits
Community Building and Social Interaction:

Group Classes: Participating in chair yoga classes provides opportunities for social interaction, fostering a sense of community and belonging. These classes can be in-person or virtual, depending on accessibility and convenience.
Shared Experiences: Engaging in chair yoga with others creates shared experiences, strengthening social bonds and creating a support network.
Support Networks and Friendships:

Building Relationships: Regular attendance at chair yoga classes can lead to lasting friendships and support networks, reducing feelings of loneliness and isolation.
Mutual Support: Practicing chair yoga in a group setting encourages mutual support and encouragement, enhancing the overall experience and commitment to the practice.
Social Engagement and Activities:

Participation in Events: Chair yoga often includes social events and activities, such as workshops, retreats, and community gatherings. These events provide additional opportunities for social engagement and connection.
Volunteer and Leadership Opportunities: Advanced practitioners of chair yoga may have opportunities to volunteer or take on leadership roles within the community, further enhancing social engagement and fulfillment.
Improved Communication and Empathy:

Enhanced Listening Skills: Mindfulness practices in chair yoga improve listening skills and presence, leading to better communication with others.
Increased Empathy: Chair yoga fosters empathy by encouraging practitioners to be present and aware of their own emotions and the emotions of others, enhancing interpersonal relationships.
Examples of Chair Yoga Practices for Emotional and Social Benefits
Emotional Benefits:

Breath Awareness: Sit comfortably with eyes closed, focusing on the breath. Practice deep, slow breathing for several minutes to calm the mind and reduce stress.
Heart-Opening Pose: Sit with your back straight, clasp your hands behind your back, and gently lift your chest. This pose can help release emotional tension and promote a sense of openness.
Social Benefits:

Partner Stretches: In a class setting, practice gentle partner stretches that encourage cooperation and connection. For example, sit facing a partner, hold each other's forearms, and take turns leaning back for a supported stretch.

Group Meditation: End a chair yoga session with a group meditation, sitting in a circle and focusing on collective breathing and presence. This fosters a sense of unity and shared experience.

Conclusion

Chair yoga offers profound emotional and social benefits that contribute to a well-rounded and fulfilling life. By reducing stress, enhancing emotional regulation, and promoting social connections, chair yoga supports overall well-being. Practicing chair yoga regularly can lead to a happier, more connected, and emotionally balanced life, making it a valuable addition to the routines of seniors and individuals with limited mobility. Embracing these benefits can transform not only your own life but also the lives of those around you, fostering a supportive and connected community.

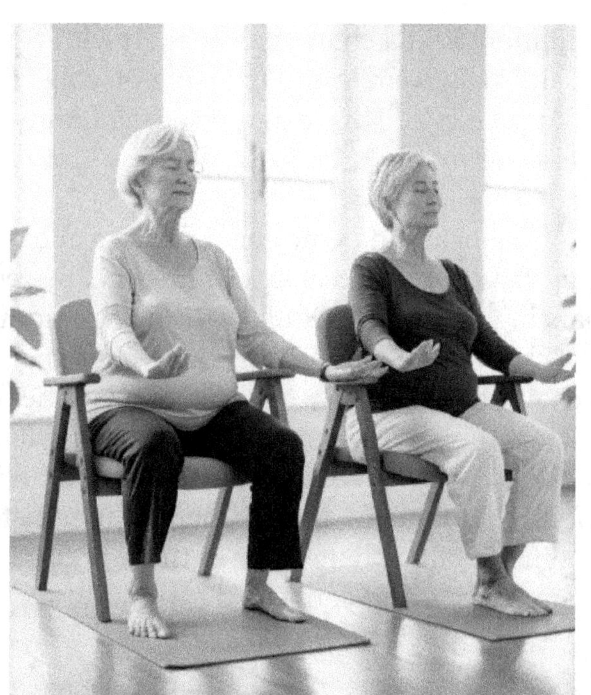

Chapter 11: Getting Started

Embarking on your chair yoga journey is an exciting step towards improving your physical, mental, and emotional well-being. This chapter will guide you through the essential preparations and considerations to ensure a safe and effective practice.

Consulting Your Doctor
Importance of Medical Advice Before Starting:

Personalized Health Assessment: Before beginning chair yoga, it's crucial to consult with your healthcare provider to assess your overall health and identify any specific conditions or limitations that may affect your practice.
Safety First: Your doctor can provide guidance on any modifications or precautions needed to ensure that your practice is safe and beneficial.
Key Questions to Ask Your Healthcare Provider:

Physical Limitations: Are there any movements or positions I should avoid due to my health conditions?
Medications: Could my current medications affect my ability to practice yoga safely?
Health Goals: How can chair yoga support my specific health goals, such as improving mobility or managing pain?
Choosing the Right Chair
Characteristics of an Ideal Chair for Chair Yoga:

Sturdy and Stable: Ensure the chair is sturdy and does not wobble. A chair with a firm, flat seat and a straight back is ideal.
No Armrests (Optional): While armrests can provide support, a chair without armrests allows for a greater range of motion and flexibility in poses.

Proper Height: The chair should be high enough so that your feet can rest flat on the floor with your knees at a 90-degree angle.
Safety Tips:

Non-Slip Surface: Place the chair on a non-slip surface or use a yoga mat to prevent slipping.
Check Stability: Always check the chair for stability before starting your practice.
Avoid Rolling Chairs: Use a stationary chair rather than one with wheels to prevent accidents.
Setting Up Your Space
Creating a Safe and Comfortable Environment:

Quiet Area: Choose a quiet, peaceful area where you won't be disturbed during your practice.
Adequate Space: Ensure there is enough space around the chair to move freely and safely.
Necessary Equipment and Props:

Yoga Straps: These can help with stretching and maintaining proper alignment in poses.
Blocks: Yoga blocks can provide support and stability, especially in deeper stretches.
Cushions and Blankets: Use these for added comfort and support, particularly for seated or reclining poses.
Establishing a Routine
Consistency is Key:

Set a Schedule: Decide on a regular time for your chair yoga practice to build a consistent routine. Even short, daily sessions can be highly beneficial.
Start Slowly: Begin with shorter sessions and gradually increase the duration and intensity as you become more comfortable and confident.
Staying Motivated:

Track Progress: Keep a journal to track your progress and note any improvements in flexibility, strength, and overall well-being.

Join a Class: Consider joining a chair yoga class, either in-person or online, to stay motivated and connected with others.

Conclusion

Starting your chair yoga journey requires some preparation and consideration, but the benefits are well worth the effort. By consulting with your doctor, choosing the right chair, setting up a safe and comfortable space, and establishing a routine, you can ensure a successful and rewarding practice. Embrace the journey with patience and openness, and you'll soon experience the numerous physical, mental, and emotional benefits of chair yoga.

Chapter 12: Consulting Your Doctor

Before beginning any new exercise regimen, especially if you have underlying health conditions or are over 60, it's crucial to consult with your healthcare provider. This chapter will guide you through the importance of seeking medical advice, the key questions to ask your doctor, and how to use this information to practice chair yoga safely and effectively.

Importance of Medical Advice Before Starting
Personal Health Assessment:

Comprehensive Evaluation: A visit to your healthcare provider allows for a thorough evaluation of your overall health status. This ensures that you understand any limitations or special considerations related to your condition. Customized Guidance: Your doctor can provide specific recommendations tailored to your health needs, helping to avoid any potential risks associated with physical activity. Prevention of Injuries:

Identifying Contraindications: Certain health conditions, such as severe osteoporosis, heart disease, or recent surgeries, may require modifications or avoidance of specific movements. Your doctor can identify these and advise accordingly. Safe Exercise Parameters: Understanding your safe heart rate range, blood pressure limits, and other vital parameters can help you exercise safely without overexertion. Key Questions to Ask Your Healthcare Provider Physical Limitations:

Movement Restrictions: Are there specific movements or positions I should avoid due to my health conditions?
Impact of Existing Conditions: How might my existing conditions (e.g., arthritis, diabetes) affect my ability to practice yoga?
Medications:

Side Effects and Exercise: Could my current medications affect my ability to practice yoga safely? Are there any side effects that I should be aware of during physical activity?
Timing of Medication: Is there an optimal time to practice yoga in relation to my medication schedule?
Health Goals:

Exercise Recommendations: How can chair yoga support my specific health goals, such as improving mobility, managing pain, or enhancing cardiovascular health?
Monitoring Progress: What signs should I look for to gauge whether the exercise is beneficial or if I need to adjust my routine?
Using Medical Advice to Guide Your Practice
Developing a Personalized Plan:

Collaborate with Your Doctor: Use the information provided by your healthcare provider to develop a chair yoga plan that aligns with your health needs and goals.
Start Slowly: Begin with gentle movements and short sessions, gradually increasing as advised by your doctor.
Adjusting Your Routine:

Modifications: Implement any recommended modifications to poses or routines to ensure they are safe and effective for your condition.
Monitoring Symptoms: Keep track of how your body responds to the practice. Note any discomfort, pain, or unusual symptoms and discuss them with your doctor.

Regular Check-Ins:

Follow-Up Visits: Schedule regular follow-up visits with your healthcare provider to monitor your progress and make any necessary adjustments to your exercise plan.
Feedback Loop: Provide feedback to your doctor about your yoga practice, including any benefits you're experiencing or challenges you're facing. This helps refine your plan for optimal results.
Conclusion
Consulting your doctor before starting chair yoga is a crucial step in ensuring a safe and effective practice. By obtaining personalized medical advice, asking the right questions, and using this guidance to tailor your yoga routine, you can confidently embark on your chair yoga journey. This proactive approach helps prevent injuries, addresses specific health concerns, and enhances the overall benefits of your practice, contributing to a healthier and more active lifestyle.

Chapter 12: Importance of Medical Advice Before Starting

Before embarking on any new exercise program, particularly for seniors and those with existing health conditions, it's crucial to consult with a healthcare provider. This chapter will delve into why seeking medical advice is essential, the benefits of doing so, and how it can help tailor a safe and effective chair yoga practice.

Comprehensive Health Evaluation
Understanding Your Health Status:

Detailed Health Assessment: A visit to your healthcare provider allows for a comprehensive assessment of your overall health. This includes evaluating any chronic conditions, current medications, and overall physical fitness. Identifying Risk Factors: Your doctor can identify specific risk factors or conditions that might affect your ability to practice chair yoga safely. This could include heart disease, osteoporosis, arthritis, or balance issues.
Personalized Recommendations:

Tailored Advice: Healthcare providers can offer personalized recommendations based on your health status. This ensures that your chair yoga practice is customized to your individual needs and limitations.
Preventing Complications: By understanding your specific health concerns, your doctor can help prevent complications that might arise from certain poses or movements.
Prevention of Injuries

Safety First:

Avoiding Harmful Movements: Some yoga poses may not be suitable for individuals with certain health conditions. For instance, those with severe osteoporosis might need to avoid forward bends to prevent fractures. Your doctor can advise on which movements to avoid.

Safe Exercise Parameters: Knowing your safe heart rate range, blood pressure limits, and other health metrics helps ensure that you exercise within safe boundaries, reducing the risk of overexertion or injury.

Adaptations and Modifications:

Recommended Adjustments: Your doctor can suggest specific adaptations or modifications to standard yoga poses that make them safer and more accessible. This ensures that you can participate fully without putting yourself at risk.

Using Props: Recommendations might include the use of props like yoga straps, blocks, or cushions to provide support and stability, making exercises safer and more comfortable.

Maximizing Health Benefits

Enhanced Effectiveness:

Targeted Health Goals: Consulting with your healthcare provider can help you set realistic and achievable health goals. Whether it's improving flexibility, managing pain, or enhancing cardiovascular health, your doctor can guide you on how chair yoga can help meet these goals.

Monitoring Progress: Regular check-ins with your healthcare provider can help monitor your progress and adjust your practice as needed. This ensures that you are continually moving towards your health objectives.

Integrated Health Management:

Holistic Approach: Combining chair yoga with other aspects of your health management plan, such as medication, diet, and other exercises, provides a holistic approach to well-being. Your doctor can help integrate these elements effectively.

Feedback Loop: Continuous feedback from your yoga practice can inform your healthcare provider about what works best for you, allowing for ongoing adjustments and improvements to your routine.

Psychological Reassurance

Building Confidence:

Peace of Mind: Knowing that a healthcare professional has reviewed and approved your exercise plan can provide significant peace of mind. This reassurance can boost your confidence and motivation to practice regularly.

Informed Decisions: Understanding the medical reasoning behind certain recommendations helps you make informed decisions about your health and exercise routine.

Encouragement and Support:

Professional Support: Having the support of a healthcare provider can encourage you to stick with your practice, knowing that it is beneficial and safe. This support can be crucial, especially when starting a new exercise regimen.

Addressing Concerns: If you experience any issues or concerns during your practice, having a healthcare provider to consult with can provide timely advice and solutions, keeping your practice safe and effective.

Conclusion

Seeking medical advice before starting chair yoga is an essential step in ensuring a safe, effective, and personalized practice. By understanding your health status, preventing injuries, maximizing benefits, and gaining psychological reassurance, you can confidently embark on your chair yoga journey. This proactive approach not only safeguards your health but also enhances the overall experience, helping you achieve a balanced and fulfilling lifestyle through the practice of chair yoga.

Chapter 13: Key Questions to Ask Your Healthcare Provider

Before beginning your chair yoga journey, it's important to have a thorough conversation with your healthcare provider. This chapter provides a comprehensive list of questions to help you gather essential information and ensure your practice is safe and tailored to your needs.

Physical Limitations
Movement Restrictions:

Are there specific movements or positions I should avoid due to my health conditions?
This question helps identify any yoga poses or movements that might aggravate existing conditions, such as arthritis or osteoporosis.
Are there any activities or exercises I should focus on to improve my specific health issues?
Understanding what exercises can benefit your specific condition can help tailor your yoga routine to your needs.
Impact of Existing Conditions:

How might my existing conditions (e.g., arthritis, diabetes) affect my ability to practice yoga?
Knowing the impact of your health conditions on yoga practice ensures that you can modify poses and routines to suit your needs.
What precautions should I take due to my current health conditions?
This question helps identify any extra measures you need to take to practice safely, such as using props or avoiding certain poses.

Medications
Side Effects and Exercise:

Could my current medications affect my ability to practice
yoga safely?
Some medications may have side effects that impact your
balance, heart rate, or energy levels, which can affect your
yoga practice.
Are there any side effects that I should be aware of during
physical activity?
Understanding potential side effects helps you stay alert to
any symptoms that may arise during your practice.
Timing of Medication:

Is there an optimal time to practice yoga in relation to my
medication schedule?
Certain medications may require you to adjust the timing of
your exercise routine. For example, you might need to avoid
practicing yoga immediately after taking medications that
cause drowsiness or affect your balance.
Should I monitor any specific health metrics (e.g., blood sugar
levels) during my practice?
This question is particularly important for conditions like
diabetes, where monitoring blood sugar levels can help
prevent hypoglycemia during exercise.
Health Goals
Exercise Recommendations:

How can chair yoga support my specific health goals, such as
improving mobility, managing pain, or enhancing
cardiovascular health?
This question helps you understand how chair yoga can be an
effective part of your health management plan.
What are realistic expectations for my progress and benefits
from practicing chair yoga?

Setting realistic expectations ensures that you stay motivated and focused on achievable goals.
Monitoring Progress:

What signs should I look for to gauge whether the exercise is beneficial or if I need to adjust my routine?
Knowing what positive signs to look for, as well as any red flags, helps you monitor your progress and make necessary adjustments.
How often should I follow up with you to review my progress and any concerns?
Regular check-ins with your healthcare provider ensure that your yoga practice continues to be safe and effective.
Safety Precautions
Emergency Protocols:

What should I do if I experience pain or discomfort during my practice?
Knowing how to respond to pain or discomfort can prevent injuries and ensure that you practice safely.
Are there any signs or symptoms that would require me to stop immediately and seek medical attention?
Identifying serious symptoms that require immediate attention helps you stay safe during your practice.
Special Equipment:

Would you recommend any specific equipment or props to support my practice?
Using the right equipment can enhance your practice by providing additional support and safety.
Are there any specific modifications you recommend for my practice?
Custom modifications ensure that your yoga routine is tailored to your abilities and health needs.
Integrating Chair Yoga into Your Routine
Complementary Activities:

Can chair yoga be integrated with other forms of exercise I'm currently doing?
Understanding how chair yoga fits into your overall exercise routine ensures a balanced and comprehensive approach to fitness.
Are there any other activities or lifestyle changes you recommend to complement my yoga practice?
Complementary activities and lifestyle changes can enhance the benefits of your yoga practice and overall well-being.
Consistency and Frequency:

How often should I practice chair yoga to see meaningful benefits?
Knowing the recommended frequency helps you establish a consistent practice routine.
Should I start with shorter sessions and gradually increase the duration?
Gradual progression ensures that you build strength and flexibility safely over time.
Conclusion
Asking these key questions during your consultation with your healthcare provider will help you gather the necessary information to start your chair yoga practice safely and effectively. By understanding your physical limitations, the impact of medications, and how to align your practice with your health goals, you can embark on your yoga journey with confidence and peace of mind. This proactive approach ensures that your chair yoga routine is not only safe but also tailored to enhance your overall well-being.

Chapter 14: Choosing the Right Chair

Selecting the appropriate chair for your chair yoga practice is crucial to ensure comfort, stability, and safety. This chapter will guide you through the characteristics to look for in an ideal chair, safety considerations, and how to set up your chair yoga space effectively.

Characteristics of an Ideal Chair for Chair Yoga
Sturdy and Stable:

Solid Construction: Choose a chair with a sturdy frame that can support your weight without wobbling or tipping over.
Flat, Firm Seat: Opt for a chair with a flat seat that provides a stable surface for seated poses and movements.
Back Support:

Straight Back: A chair with a straight back offers good support for your spine during upright poses and ensures proper alignment.
No Armrests (Optional): While armrests can provide additional support, consider a chair without armrests to allow for more freedom of movement in certain poses.
Height Considerations:

Adjustable Height: If possible, choose a chair with adjustable height settings to accommodate different body sizes and leg lengths.

Feet Flat on Floor: Ensure that when seated, your feet can rest flat on the floor with your knees at a 90-degree angle for optimal stability and comfort.

Safety Tips

Non-Slip Surface:

Place on a Stable Surface: Position the chair on a non-slip surface such as a yoga mat or carpet to prevent it from sliding during movements.

Check Stability: Before starting your practice, check that the chair is stable and secure to avoid accidents or falls.

Avoid Rolling Chairs:

Stationary Chair: Use a stationary chair rather than one with wheels to prevent unexpected movement and ensure stability during poses.

Setting Up Your Chair Yoga Space

Clear, Open Area:

Ample Space Around the Chair: Choose a location with enough room around the chair to comfortably extend your arms and legs during poses.

Quiet Environment: Select a quiet space where you can focus without distractions, enhancing your yoga experience.

Equipment and Props:

Yoga Props: Gather necessary props such as yoga straps, blocks, and cushions to support and enhance your practice.

Storage: Keep your props nearby for easy access during your yoga sessions.

Personalizing Your Chair Yoga Practice

Customizing Your Setup:

Chair Positioning: Experiment with the chair's positioning to find what feels most comfortable and supportive for your body.

Modifications: Make adjustments as needed, such as using cushions or blankets to modify the seat or backrest for added comfort and support.
Adapting Poses:

Use of Props: Incorporate props to assist in achieving proper alignment and deepen stretches without straining muscles or joints.
Modify Intensity: Adjust the intensity of poses by modifying the range of motion or duration based on your comfort level and physical ability.
Conclusion
Choosing the right chair for your chair yoga practice involves selecting a sturdy, stable chair with appropriate back support and adjustable height options. Ensuring a safe setup with a non-slip surface and adequate space around the chair enhances your comfort and allows for a more focused and effective practice. By personalizing your chair yoga space and making use of props as needed, you can create a supportive environment that promotes relaxation, flexibility, and overall well-being during your yoga sessions.

Chapter 15: Characteristics of an Ideal Chair for Chair Yoga

Selecting the right chair is fundamental to ensuring a safe and effective chair yoga practice, especially for seniors and individuals with physical limitations. This chapter explores the key characteristics that make a chair suitable for chair yoga, focusing on stability, support, and adaptability to different body types and needs.

Stability and Durability
Sturdy Frame:

Solid Construction: Choose a chair with a sturdy frame that can support your weight and provide stability during various yoga poses.
No Wobbling: Ensure the chair does not wobble or sway, especially when performing movements that require balance.
Non-Slip Feet:

Floor Grips: Opt for chairs with rubber or non-slip feet to prevent sliding or shifting during yoga sessions, enhancing safety and stability.
Seat and Back Support
Flat Seat Surface:

Firm and Level: Select a chair with a flat, firm seat surface to support seated poses comfortably. This provides a stable foundation for exercises and ensures proper alignment.
Straight Backrest:

Optimal Support: Look for chairs with a straight backrest that promotes good posture and spine alignment. This supports the back during upright poses and reduces strain.
Height Adjustability
Adjustable Height:

Versatility: Choose a chair with adjustable height settings to accommodate different body sizes and preferences. This allows for customization to achieve optimal comfort and alignment.
Feet Placement: When seated, ensure your feet can rest flat on the floor with knees bent at a 90-degree angle for stability and proper posture.
Armrest Considerations
Optional Armrests:

Freedom of Movement: Consider chairs with removable or optional armrests to allow for more freedom of movement during yoga poses that require arm extension.
Accessibility: Armrests can provide additional support for those who may need assistance getting in and out of the chair or during seated poses.
Accessibility and Comfort
Ease of Use:

Accessible Design: Choose a chair that is easy to get into and out of, especially for individuals with mobility challenges.
Comfort Features: Look for features like padded seats or cushions that enhance comfort during prolonged sitting or when holding poses.
Conclusion

Selecting an ideal chair for chair yoga involves prioritizing stability, support, and adaptability to accommodate your unique needs and preferences. By choosing a chair with a sturdy frame, non-slip features, appropriate seat and back support, adjustable height options, and optional armrests, you can create a safe and comfortable environment for your chair yoga practice. These characteristics not only enhance your ability to perform yoga poses effectively but also contribute to a positive and enjoyable yoga experience that promotes relaxation, flexibility, and overall well-being.

Chapter 16: Safety Tips for Chair Yoga Practice

Safety is paramount when practicing chair yoga, especially for seniors and individuals with physical limitations. This chapter outlines essential safety tips to ensure a safe and enjoyable chair yoga experience.

Setting Up Your Practice Space
Stable Surface:

Place your chair on a stable, non-slip surface such as a yoga mat or carpet to prevent it from sliding during movements.
Ample Space:

Ensure there is enough space around the chair to comfortably extend your arms and legs during poses without obstruction.
Chair Stability
Check Chair Stability:

Before starting your practice, ensure the chair is stable and secure. Check for any loose parts or instability that could affect your safety during poses.
Avoid Rolling Chairs:

Use a stationary chair rather than one with wheels to prevent unexpected movement and maintain stability during poses.
Personal Health Considerations
Consult Your Healthcare Provider:

Seek medical advice before starting chair yoga, especially if you have any pre-existing health conditions or concerns.
Listen to Your Body:

Pay attention to your body's signals during practice. If you experience pain or discomfort, modify or discontinue the pose as needed.

Movement and Poses

Modify Poses as Necessary:

Use props such as yoga blocks or cushions to modify poses and accommodate your range of motion or physical limitations.

Avoid Overexertion:

Practice within your comfort zone and avoid pushing yourself too hard. Gradually increase the intensity of poses as your strength and flexibility improve.

Breathing and Relaxation

Focus on Breathing:

Incorporate mindful breathing techniques to enhance relaxation and reduce stress during practice.

Stay Hydrated:

Drink water before and after your practice session to stay hydrated, especially if practicing for an extended period.

Conclusion

By following these safety tips, you can create a safe and supportive environment for your chair yoga practice. Prioritize stability, consult with your healthcare provider as needed, and listen to your body's cues to ensure a positive and beneficial chair yoga experience. Safety precautions not only protect you from injury but also promote confidence and enjoyment in your yoga journey, fostering improved flexibility, strength, and overall well-being.

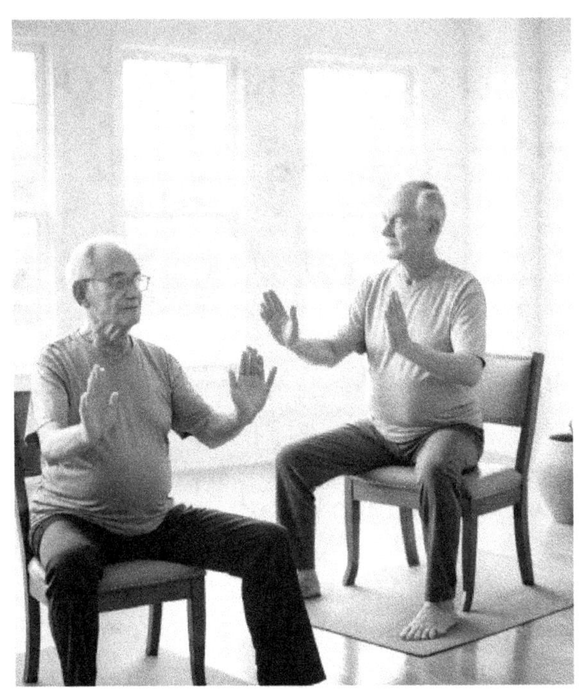

Chapter 17: Setting Up Your Chair Yoga Space

Creating a conducive environment for chair yoga is essential for a comfortable and effective practice. This chapter provides guidance on how to set up your space to enhance safety, comfort, and focus during your chair yoga sessions.

Choosing the Location
Quiet and Peaceful Environment:

Select a space that is free from distractions and noise, allowing you to focus fully on your practice.
Adequate Lighting:

Ensure the space is well-lit to prevent tripping or straining your eyes during poses and movements.
Positioning Your Chair
Stable Surface:

Place your chair on a stable surface such as a yoga mat or non-slip flooring to prevent it from moving during practice.
Ample Space Around the Chair:

Ensure there is enough room around the chair for comfortable movement and extension of your arms and legs during poses.
Gathering Equipment and Props
Essential Props:

Gather necessary props such as yoga blocks, straps, and cushions to support your practice and enhance comfort.
Accessibility:

Keep props within reach to easily access them during your session without interrupting your flow.
Creating a Supportive Atmosphere
Comfortable Temperature:

Maintain a comfortable room temperature to prevent overheating or discomfort during your practice.
Personalization:

Customize your space with calming elements such as plants, soothing music, or aromatherapy to enhance relaxation.
Safety Precautions
Clear Space:

Remove any obstacles or hazards from the area around your chair to prevent tripping or injury during poses.
Emergency Access:

Ensure that emergency exits are clear and accessible in case of any unforeseen situations.
Personal Preparation
Proper Attire:

Wear comfortable, breathable clothing that allows for ease of movement and does not restrict your range of motion.
Hydration:

Have a bottle of water nearby to stay hydrated throughout your practice, especially if engaging in longer sessions.
Conclusion

Setting up your chair yoga space thoughtfully enhances your overall practice experience, promoting safety, comfort, and focus. By choosing a quiet and well-lit location, positioning your chair on a stable surface, gathering necessary props, and personalizing your environment, you create an inviting atmosphere conducive to relaxation and mindful movement. Incorporating these elements ensures that your chair yoga sessions are enjoyable, effective, and beneficial for your physical and mental well-being.

Chapter 18: Creating a Safe and Comfortable Environment for Chair Yoga

Establishing a safe and comfortable environment is essential for a fulfilling chair yoga practice, particularly for seniors and individuals with varying physical abilities. This chapter focuses on practical strategies to ensure safety and comfort throughout your chair yoga sessions.

Safety Measures
Stable Chair Placement:

Position your chair on a flat, non-slip surface such as a yoga mat or carpet to prevent it from shifting or sliding during movements.
Check Chair Stability:

Before each session, ensure the chair is stable and all components are securely in place to avoid accidents or falls.
Clear Surroundings:

Remove obstacles or clutter around the chair to create a clear space for movement and prevent tripping hazards.
Comfort Enhancements
Supportive Seating:

Use cushions or pillows to adjust the seat and backrest of the chair for optimal comfort and posture alignment.
Appropriate Clothing:

Wear loose, comfortable clothing that allows for unrestricted movement and doesn't restrict your range of motion.
Lighting and Atmosphere
Adequate Lighting:

Ensure the space is well-lit to facilitate safe movement and prevent strain on your eyes during poses.
Temperature Control:

Maintain a comfortable room temperature to prevent overheating or discomfort during your practice.
Accessibility Considerations
Accessibility Features:

Ensure the chair and practice area are accessible for individuals with mobility challenges, allowing for easy entry and exit.
Props and Equipment:

Have necessary props such as yoga blocks, straps, and blankets nearby to support your practice and enhance comfort.
Personal Health Awareness
Hydration:

Keep a water bottle nearby to stay hydrated throughout your practice, especially important for longer sessions.
Listening to Your Body:

Pay attention to your body's signals and adjust poses or take breaks as needed to prevent overexertion or injury.
Conclusion

Creating a safe and comfortable environment for chair yoga involves thoughtful preparation and attention to detail. By implementing these strategies — ensuring chair stability, clearing the space, enhancing comfort with supportive seating and appropriate clothing, optimizing lighting and temperature, considering accessibility needs, and maintaining personal health awareness — you can cultivate an environment that supports your physical well-being and enhances your yoga practice experience. Prioritizing safety and comfort allows you to fully enjoy the benefits of chair yoga, promoting relaxation, flexibility, and overall health improvement.

Chapter 19: Necessary Equipment and Props for Chair Yoga

Choosing the right equipment and props enhances your chair yoga practice by providing support, stability, and assistance in achieving proper alignment. This chapter explores essential equipment and props that can enrich your chair yoga sessions.

Yoga Straps
Purpose:

Assist in Stretching: Yoga straps help increase flexibility by extending your reach during seated stretches and poses.
Usage:

Loop and Hold: Securely loop the strap around your foot or leg to gently deepen stretches without straining muscles or joints.
Yoga Blocks
Purpose:

Support and Stability: Yoga blocks provide height and stability for poses that require reaching the floor or modifying seated positions.
Usage:

Under Hands or Feet: Place blocks under your hands or feet to achieve proper alignment and support during poses like forward folds or seated twists.
Cushions and Bolsters
Purpose:

Comfort and Support: Cushions and bolsters provide added comfort and support, especially for individuals with limited flexibility or mobility.
Usage:

Seat and Back Support: Use cushions to modify the seat or backrest of the chair for better posture alignment and comfort during prolonged sitting.
Blankets or Towels
Purpose:

Padding and Warmth: Blankets or towels offer padding for sensitive areas and can provide warmth during relaxation poses.
Usage:

Under Knees or Seat: Fold blankets under your knees for extra cushioning or place over your legs for warmth during relaxation exercises.
Additional Props
Therabands or Resistance Bands:

Strength Building: These bands can be used to add resistance for strength-building exercises, enhancing muscle tone and flexibility.
Small Balls or Rollers:

Massage and Mobility: Use small balls or rollers to release tension in muscles and improve joint mobility during warm-up or cool-down sessions.
Conclusion

Incorporating essential equipment and props into your chair yoga practice enhances comfort, stability, and alignment, supporting your physical and mental well-being. Whether you use yoga straps for stretching, blocks for support, cushions for comfort, or other props for specific needs, these tools help customize your practice to suit your individual capabilities and goals. By integrating these props effectively, you can deepen your stretches, maintain proper alignment, and explore a variety of poses with confidence and safety, making your chair yoga experience more rewarding and beneficial overall.

Chapter 20: Chair Yoga Basics

Chair yoga offers a gentle yet effective approach to yoga practice, suitable for individuals of all ages and abilities. This chapter introduces the foundational principles and basic elements of chair yoga, providing a solid starting point for beginners and a refresher for seasoned practitioners.

Understanding Chair Yoga
Definition:

Chair yoga adapts traditional yoga poses to be performed while seated or using a chair for support. It focuses on gentle movements, stretches, and breathing exercises to promote flexibility, strength, and relaxation.
Benefits:

Accessibility: Chair yoga is accessible to seniors, individuals with mobility issues, or those recovering from injury, allowing them to enjoy the benefits of yoga in a safe and supported manner.
Improved Mobility: Regular practice can improve joint mobility, flexibility, and range of motion, enhancing overall physical function.
Stress Relief: Breathing exercises and relaxation techniques incorporated in chair yoga help reduce stress, promote mental clarity, and improve emotional well-being.
Basic Components of Chair Yoga
Breathing Techniques:

Importance: Emphasizes the connection between breath and movement. Deep, mindful breathing helps relax the body, calm the mind, and enhance focus during practice.

Techniques: Simple breathing exercises such as diaphragmatic breathing (belly breathing) or counted breaths are introduced to promote relaxation and centering.
Basic Chair Yoga Poses:

Seated Mountain Pose: Aligns the spine, improves posture, and promotes grounding and stability.
Seated Forward Fold: Stretches the back and hamstrings, encourages relaxation, and releases tension in the spine.
Seated Twist: Enhances spinal mobility, massages internal organs, and promotes detoxification.
Seated Side Stretch: Increases flexibility in the sides of the body, improves breathing capacity, and relieves tension in the shoulders and neck.
Modifications and Adaptations:

Individual Needs: Provides variations and modifications for different abilities, ensuring that poses can be adjusted to accommodate limitations or specific health conditions.
Use of Props: Introduces the use of props such as yoga blocks, straps, or cushions to assist in achieving proper alignment and support during poses.
Warm-up Exercises
Purpose:

Prepare the Body: Gentle movements and stretches to warm up muscles, lubricate joints, and increase circulation, preparing the body for deeper yoga practice.
Examples: Neck rolls, shoulder shrugs, gentle spinal twists, ankle and wrist circles, and seated cat-cow stretches.
Conclusion

Mastering the basics of chair yoga lays the foundation for a safe, enjoyable, and beneficial practice. By understanding the principles of chair yoga, including breathing techniques, basic poses, modifications for individual needs, and the importance of warm-up exercises, practitioners can build strength, flexibility, and relaxation while seated. Whether you're new to yoga or seeking a gentle alternative to traditional practice, chair yoga offers a holistic approach to wellness that can be integrated into daily life with ease and accessibility.

Chapter 21: Breathing Techniques in Chair Yoga

Breathing techniques, or pranayama, are fundamental in chair yoga practice, influencing both physical and mental well-being. This chapter explores various breathing techniques tailored for a seated practice, enhancing relaxation, focus, and overall mindfulness.

Importance of Breath in Chair Yoga
Mind-Body Connection:

Centering and Focus: Conscious breathing connects the mind and body, promoting a sense of calm and enhancing concentration during yoga poses.
Stress Reduction:

Relaxation Response: Deep, diaphragmatic breathing triggers the parasympathetic nervous system, promoting relaxation and reducing stress levels.
Simple Breathing Exercises
1. Diaphragmatic Breathing (Belly Breathing):

Technique: Inhale deeply through the nose, allowing the belly to expand outward. Exhale slowly through pursed lips, drawing the navel toward the spine.
Benefits: Increases oxygen intake, reduces tension in the chest and shoulders, and promotes relaxation.
2. Counted Breath (Box Breathing):

Technique: Inhale deeply for a count of four, hold the breath for a count of four, exhale slowly for a count of four, and hold the breath out for a count of four. Repeat in a continuous cycle.
Benefits: Enhances concentration, calms the mind, and regulates the breath cycle.
3. Equal Breathing (Sama Vritti):

Technique: Inhale for a count of four, exhale for a count of four, maintaining an equal duration for both inhalation and exhalation.
Benefits: Balances the nervous system, increases mental clarity, and promotes a sense of equilibrium.
Incorporating Breath with Movement
Syncing Breath and Movement:

Flowing Sequence: Coordinate inhalations and exhalations with gentle movements or stretches, enhancing the fluidity and mindfulness of your practice.
Breath Awareness:

Mindful Observation: Remain aware of the natural rhythm of your breath throughout the practice, using it as a guide for movement and relaxation.
Practical Tips
Comfortable Seating:

Positioning: Sit comfortably with feet flat on the floor and spine tall, allowing for unrestricted diaphragmatic movement during breathing exercises.
Consistency:

Regular Practice: Incorporate breathing techniques into daily routines to cultivate resilience to stress and enhance overall well-being.
Conclusion

Breathing techniques form a cornerstone of chair yoga practice, fostering relaxation, mental clarity, and mind-body awareness. By mastering simple yet effective techniques such as diaphragmatic breathing, counted breath, and equal breathing, practitioners can harness the transformative power of breath to support their physical and emotional health. Whether used as a standalone practice or integrated with yoga poses, these techniques provide invaluable tools for managing stress, improving focus, and nurturing a deeper connection to oneself in chair yoga practice.

Chapter 22: Importance of Breath in Chair Yoga

Breath, or prana, is integral to yoga practice, including chair yoga, as it serves as a bridge connecting the mind, body, and spirit. This chapter delves into the significance of breath and its profound impact on physical, mental, and emotional well-being within the context of chair yoga.

Mind-Body Connection
Centering and Presence:

Anchor for Awareness: Conscious breathing anchors attention to the present moment, fostering mindfulness and deepening the mind-body connection.
Enhanced Focus:

Clarity and Concentration: Breath awareness cultivates mental clarity, sharpening focus during yoga poses and daily activities.
Physiological Benefits
Regulation of Stress Response:

Activating the Relaxation Response: Deep, slow breathing stimulates the parasympathetic nervous system, promoting relaxation and reducing stress hormones like cortisol.
Oxygenation:

Improved Oxygen Intake: Deep breathing enhances oxygen flow to muscles and organs, optimizing physical performance and overall vitality.
Emotional Regulation
Stress Reduction:

Calming Effect: Mindful breathing alleviates anxiety, restlessness, and emotional turbulence, promoting a sense of calm and emotional balance.
Mood Enhancement:

Promoting Positivity: Breath practices can uplift mood, increase resilience to negative emotions, and foster a positive outlook on life.
Energizing and Relaxing Techniques
Energizing Breath (Kapalabhati):

Technique: Rapid, forceful exhalations followed by passive inhalations. Energizes the body and clears the mind.
Relaxing Breath (Nadi Shodhana):

Technique: Alternate nostril breathing, balancing the flow of energy in the body, and inducing a state of relaxation.
Integration with Movement
Flow and Fluidity:

Syncing Breath with Movement: Coordinating inhalations and exhalations with yoga poses enhances movement efficiency, grace, and mindfulness.
Breath-Centered Practices:

Breath Awareness: Cultivate awareness of the breath's natural rhythm and depth throughout chair yoga practice, using it as a guide for pacing and relaxation.
Everyday Application
Mindful Living:

Translating Practice into Daily Life: Incorporate breath awareness into daily routines to manage stress, enhance focus, and maintain emotional equilibrium.
Conclusion

The profound role of breath in chair yoga extends beyond physical exercise, encompassing mental clarity, emotional regulation, and spiritual growth. By embracing breath as a foundational element of practice, practitioners unlock its transformative potential to cultivate resilience, vitality, and inner peace. Whether engaging in energizing breath techniques to invigorate the body or soothing practices to calm the mind, integrating breath awareness into chair yoga enhances holistic well-being, supporting a balanced and harmonious lifestyle.

Chapter 23: Simple Breathing Exercises in Chair Yoga

Breathing exercises are foundational in chair yoga, offering profound benefits for relaxation, stress reduction, and overall well-being. This chapter introduces easy-to-practice breathing techniques tailored for seated positions, enhancing mindfulness and promoting inner calm.

Diaphragmatic Breathing (Belly Breathing)
Technique:

Sit comfortably with feet flat on the floor and hands resting on the abdomen.
Inhale deeply through the nose, allowing the belly to expand outward.
Exhale slowly through pursed lips, drawing the navel toward the spine.
Benefits:

Promotes relaxation by activating the parasympathetic nervous system.
Improves oxygenation of the body, reducing stress and anxiety levels.
Equal Breathing (Sama Vritti)
Technique:

Inhale through the nose for a count of four.
Exhale through the nose for a count of four.
Maintain equal duration for both inhalation and exhalation.
Benefits:

Balances the nervous system and calms the mind.

Enhances concentration and focus during yoga practice.
Counted Breath (Box Breathing)
Technique:

Inhale deeply through the nose for a count of four.
Hold the breath for a count of four.
Exhale slowly through the nose for a count of four.
Hold the breath out for a count of four before inhaling again.
Benefits:

Induces relaxation and reduces stress levels.
Helps regulate the breath cycle and stabilize emotions.
Alternate Nostril Breathing (Nadi Shodhana)
Technique:

Sit comfortably with spine tall and left hand resting on the
knee.
Use the right thumb to close the right nostril and inhale
deeply through the left nostril.
Close the left nostril with the right ring finger and release the
right nostril to exhale.
Inhale through the right nostril, then close it and release the
left to exhale.
Continue this alternate pattern for several rounds, focusing on
smooth, even breaths.
Benefits:

Balances the flow of energy (prana) in the body.
Clears the mind, promotes concentration, and relieves stress.
Conclusion

These simple breathing exercises form the cornerstone of chair yoga practice, offering immediate benefits for relaxation, stress relief, and mental clarity. By incorporating diaphragmatic breathing, equal breathing, counted breath, and alternate nostril breathing into your daily routine, you can cultivate a profound sense of well-being and enhance your chair yoga experience. Regular practice of these techniques empowers you to harness the transformative power of breath, promoting physical health, emotional balance, and inner peace in your journey toward holistic wellness.

Chapter 24: Basic Postures in Chair Yoga

Chair yoga incorporates a variety of basic postures designed to improve flexibility, strength, and balance while seated or using a chair for support. This chapter introduces fundamental chair yoga poses, providing clear instructions and modifications for practitioners of all abilities.

Seated Mountain Pose (Tadasana)
Technique:

Sit tall with feet flat on the floor, hip-width apart.
Align shoulders over hips, spine elongated, and hands resting gently on thighs or knees.
Close eyes if comfortable, focus on deep, steady breaths.
Benefits:

Improves posture and alignment.
Promotes grounding and centering.
Seated Forward Fold (Paschimottanasana)
Technique:

Sit tall with feet flat on the floor, legs extended in front.
Inhale, lengthen spine; exhale, hinge at hips to fold forward.
Rest hands on legs, ankles, or shins, keeping spine straight.
Hold for several breaths, release with each exhale.
Benefits:

Stretches hamstrings, lower back, and spine.
Calms the mind and relieves stress.
Seated Twist (Ardha Matsyendrasana)
Technique:

Sit tall with feet flat, spine elongated.
Inhale, lengthen spine; exhale, twist torso to the right.
Place left hand on right knee, right hand on chair back or armrest.
Hold for several breaths, then repeat on the other side.
Benefits:

Increases spinal mobility and flexibility.
Massages internal organs, improves digestion.
Seated Side Stretch (Parsva Sukhasana)
Technique:

Sit tall with feet flat, spine lengthened.
Inhale, raise left arm overhead, exhale, lean to the right.
Keep left hip grounded, avoid collapsing into the right side.
Hold for several breaths, then switch sides.
Benefits:

Stretches the sides of the torso and arms.
Improves breathing capacity and posture.
Modified Warrior II (Virabhadrasana II)
Technique:

Sit tall with feet flat, extend right leg forward.
Inhale, lift arms to shoulder height; exhale, turn torso to the right.
Bend right knee over ankle, extend left leg behind for balance.
Hold for several breaths, then switch sides.
Benefits:

Strengthens legs, improves balance.
Builds stamina and concentration.
Conclusion

These basic chair yoga postures provide a solid foundation for building strength, flexibility, and balance while seated or using a chair for support. Practicing these poses regularly enhances physical well-being, promotes relaxation, and cultivates mindfulness. Modify each posture as needed to suit individual abilities and comfort levels, ensuring a safe and enjoyable chair yoga practice that supports your journey toward holistic health and wellness.

Chapter 25: Step-by-Step Instructions for Basic Chair Yoga Poses

This chapter provides detailed instructions for essential chair yoga poses, designed to promote flexibility, strength, and relaxation. Each pose is adapted for seated practice, ensuring accessibility and safety for practitioners of all abilities.

1. Seated Mountain Pose (Tadasana)
Technique:

Sit tall with feet flat on the floor, hip-width apart.
Align shoulders over hips, spine elongated, and hands resting gently on thighs or knees.
Close eyes if comfortable, focus on deep, steady breaths.
Hold the pose for 30 seconds to 1 minute, maintaining awareness of alignment and breath.
Benefits:

Improves posture and alignment.
Promotes grounding and centering.
2. Seated Forward Fold (Paschimottanasana)
Technique:

Sit tall with feet flat on the floor, legs extended in front.
Inhale, lengthen spine; exhale, hinge at hips to fold forward.
Rest hands on legs, ankles, or shins, keeping spine straight.
Hold the stretch for 30 seconds to 1 minute, breathing deeply and releasing tension with each exhale.
Inhale to lift back to sitting position.
Benefits:

Stretches hamstrings, lower back, and spine.
Calms the mind and relieves stress.
3. Seated Twist (Ardha Matsyendrasana)
Technique:

Sit tall with feet flat on the floor, spine elongated.
Inhale, lengthen spine; exhale, twist torso to the right.
Place left hand on right knee, right hand on chair back or
armrest for support.
Hold the twist for 30 seconds to 1 minute, breathing deeply.
Inhale to release and repeat on the other side.
Benefits:

Increases spinal mobility and flexibility.
Massages internal organs, improves digestion.
4. Seated Side Stretch (Parsva Sukhasana)
Technique:

Sit tall with feet flat on the floor, spine lengthened.
Inhale, raise left arm overhead; exhale, lean to the right.
Keep left hip grounded, avoid collapsing into the right side.
Hold the stretch for 30 seconds to 1 minute, breathing deeply.
Inhale to lift back to center, then switch sides.
Benefits:

Stretches the sides of the torso and arms.
Improves breathing capacity and posture.
5. Modified Warrior II (Virabhadrasana II)
Technique:

Sit tall with feet flat on the floor, extend right leg forward.
Inhale, lift arms to shoulder height; exhale, turn torso to the
right.
Bend right knee over ankle, extend left leg behind for balance.
Hold the pose for 30 seconds to 1 minute, breathing deeply.

Inhale to lift back to center, then switch sides.
Benefits:

Strengthens legs and improves balance.
Builds stamina and concentration.
Conclusion
These step-by-step instructions for basic chair yoga poses provide a foundation for improving physical well-being, enhancing flexibility, strength, and relaxation. Practice each pose mindfully, focusing on proper alignment, breath awareness, and listening to your body's cues. Modify poses as needed to suit your comfort and abilities, ensuring a safe and enjoyable chair yoga practice that supports your journey toward holistic health and wellness.

Alignment and Posture:

Correct Alignment: Ensure you align your body properly by sitting tall with feet flat on the floor, hips-width apart. Keep your spine elongated, shoulders relaxed, and engage your core gently. This alignment helps in maintaining stability and prevents strain.
Discomfort or Strain: If you feel discomfort or strain, it's important to listen to your body. Ease out of the pose slightly, adjust your posture, or use props like cushions or blocks for support. Never force a pose beyond your comfort level.
Breathing Techniques:

Coordination with Movement: Coordinating breath with movement enhances the flow and effectiveness of chair yoga poses. Inhale during movements that expand the chest or lengthen the spine, and exhale during movements that contract or fold forward. This synchronization calms the mind and improves oxygen flow.
Specific Techniques: While basic poses generally benefit from steady, deep breathing, you can enhance relaxation with techniques like diaphragmatic breathing (deep belly breaths) or counted breath (equal inhales and exhales). Experiment with different techniques to find what feels most natural and calming for you.
Modifications and Adaptations:

Limited Mobility: Modify poses by using a higher chair or adding cushions for support. For example, in Seated Forward Fold, rest your hands on your thighs instead of reaching for your ankles if flexibility is limited.

Wheelchair Users: Adapt poses by performing upper body movements, such as seated twists or arm stretches. Focus on engaging muscles and maintaining alignment suited to your seated position.
Duration and Repetition:

Holding Poses: Aim to hold each pose for 30 seconds to 1 minute, focusing on steady breath and maintaining proper alignment. Gradually increase holding time as your flexibility and comfort level improve.
Sequence: You can repeat poses in a sequence that flows naturally for you. Start with warm-up poses like Seated Mountain Pose, move to more active poses like Seated Forward Fold or Modified Warrior II, and end with relaxing poses like Seated Twist or Seated Side Stretch.
Progression and Advancement:

Progression: As you become comfortable with basic chair yoga poses, challenge yourself by exploring more advanced variations or holding poses for longer durations. Gradually introduce new poses that build on foundational ones, such as adding a gentle backbend or incorporating balance challenges.
Additional Poses: Explore poses like Cat-Cow Stretch (Marjaryasana-Bitilasana) for spinal flexibility or Eagle Arms (Garudasana Arms) for shoulder opening, based on your increasing comfort and ability levels.
Safety and Precautions:

Consultation: It's advisable to consult with a healthcare provider before starting chair yoga, especially if you have any medical conditions or concerns. They can provide personalized recommendations and ensure chair yoga is safe and beneficial for you.

Safety Tips: Always practice within your comfort zone and avoid pushing yourself into painful positions. Use props as needed to support your body and maintain stability. If you experience dizziness, shortness of breath, or discomfort, pause and rest before continuing.

Integration into Daily Routine:

Frequency: Practice chair yoga poses daily or several times a week to experience noticeable improvements in flexibility, strength, and relaxation. Consistency is key to reaping the full benefits of yoga practice.

Incorporation: Integrate poses into your daily routine by setting aside dedicated time, such as morning stretches or midday breaks. Even short sessions can contribute to enhanced well-being and mental clarity throughout the day.

Additional Resources:

Information and Videos: Look for reputable sources that offer instructional videos or online classes specifically tailored to chair yoga. Websites of yoga organizations, reputable yoga instructors, or specialized yoga platforms often provide comprehensive resources.

Recommended Reading: Explore books and articles focused on chair yoga, which may include detailed pose descriptions, modifications, and additional tips for enhancing your practice.

Chapter 26: Modifications for Different Ability Levels in Chair Yoga

This chapter focuses on providing modifications and adaptations for chair yoga poses to accommodate practitioners with varying abilities and needs. These modifications ensure that everyone can participate in and benefit from chair yoga, regardless of physical condition or limitations.

1. Seated Mountain Pose (Tadasana)
Beginner Modification:

Sit tall with feet flat on the floor, hip-width apart.
Rest hands gently on thighs or knees.
Focus on elongating the spine and relaxing the shoulders.
Intermediate Modification:

Elevate arms slightly away from the body, palms facing forward.
Engage core muscles gently to enhance stability and alignment.
Advanced Modification:

Lift arms overhead, palms together (if comfortable).

Press feet into the floor for grounding, maintaining steady breath.

2. Seated Forward Fold (Paschimottanasana)
Beginner Modification:

Sit tall with legs extended in front, feet hip-width apart.
Rest hands on thighs, shins, or ankles for support.
Focus on lengthening the spine while gently folding forward.
Intermediate Modification:

Use a strap or belt around the feet to assist in reaching forward.
Maintain a slight bend in the knees if hamstring flexibility is limited.
Advanced Modification:

Hold onto the feet or ankles with both hands, deepening the stretch.
Keep the spine straight and engage core muscles to support the fold.

3. Seated Twist (Ardha Matsyendrasana)
Beginner Modification:

Sit tall with feet flat on the floor, spine elongated.
Place one hand on the opposite knee, gently twist torso.
Use the other hand for support on the chair armrest or back.
Intermediate Modification:

Place both hands on the outside of the opposite thigh for a deeper twist.
Keep the gaze soft and maintain steady breath throughout the twist.
Advanced Modification:

Extend the arm behind the back to reach for the chair back or opposite hip.

Deepen the twist by engaging core muscles and rotating from the base of the spine.
4. Seated Side Stretch (Parsva Sukhasana)
Beginner Modification:

Sit tall with feet flat on the floor, arms relaxed at sides.
Inhale, raise one arm overhead; exhale, lean gently to the side.
Keep opposite hand grounded on the chair seat or armrest for support.
Intermediate Modification:

Extend both arms overhead, palms facing each other.
Engage core muscles to stabilize the torso while deepening the stretch.
Advanced Modification:

Hold one wrist with the opposite hand overhead, gently pulling to deepen the stretch.
Maintain equal weight distribution through the sit bones and keep the spine lengthened.
5. Modified Warrior II (Virabhadrasana II)
Beginner Modification:

Sit tall with feet flat on the floor, extend one leg forward slightly.
Inhale, raise arms to shoulder height; exhale, turn torso to the side.
Bend the front knee slightly over the ankle, maintaining stability.
Intermediate Modification:

Ground the feet firmly into the floor for stability.
Rotate the torso further to deepen the stretch, keeping shoulders relaxed.
Advanced Modification:

Lift the back leg slightly off the floor for balance challenge. Hold the pose longer while maintaining steady breath and focused gaze.

Conclusion

These modifications for different ability levels ensure that chair yoga poses are accessible and beneficial for practitioners of all ages and physical conditions. Whether you're a beginner looking to improve flexibility or an advanced practitioner seeking to deepen your practice, these adaptations allow you to customize your chair yoga experience. Always listen to your body, honor its limitations, and gradually progress as you build strength, flexibility, and mindfulness through regular practice.

Understanding Modifications:

How do I determine which modification is appropriate for my current ability level?
Can I mix and match modifications for different poses based on how I feel each day?
Progression and Advancement:

Once I start with a beginner modification, how do I progress to intermediate or advanced levels?
Are there signs or benchmarks to look for to know when I'm ready to advance to the next level of modification?
Safety and Alignment:

How can I ensure I'm maintaining proper alignment while using modifications?
Are there specific safety considerations I should keep in mind when trying different modifications?
Incorporating Modifications into Practice:

Should I focus on mastering one modification before trying others, or can I experiment with different options during each practice session?
How can I seamlessly transition between modifications during a chair yoga session without disrupting the flow?
Personalization of Practice:

How can I tailor modifications to address specific areas of concern or limitations in my body?
Are there resources or guides that provide additional modifications beyond those mentioned in the chapter?
Feedback and Progress Tracking:

Is it beneficial to seek feedback from a yoga instructor or healthcare provider on my use of modifications?
What are effective ways to track my progress when using modifications over time?
Integration with Other Forms of Exercise:

Can I combine chair yoga modifications with other forms of exercise or physical therapy routines?
Are there specific modifications that complement activities like walking or strength training?
Long-Term Practice Goals:

How can I set realistic goals for improving flexibility, strength, and overall well-being using modifications?
What role do modifications play in maintaining a consistent chair yoga practice over the long term?

Understanding Modifications:

Determining Appropriate Modifications: Choose a modification based on your current physical abilities and comfort level. Start with the beginner modification for poses and gradually progress to intermediate or advanced as you feel more confident and comfortable.

Mixing and Matching Modifications: Yes, you can mix and match modifications based on how your body feels each day. Listen to your body's cues and select modifications that support your needs during each session. For example, you might use a deeper twist modification on days when you feel more flexible and a gentler version on days when you need more support.

Progression and Advancement:

Progressing to Higher Levels: Begin with the beginner modifications to establish foundational alignment and comfort. As you gain strength, flexibility, and confidence, gradually explore intermediate and advanced modifications. Signs of readiness include feeling stable and secure in the pose, maintaining steady breath, and being able to hold the pose comfortably for the recommended duration.

Benchmarks for Advancement: Look for improvements in flexibility, balance, and ease of movement as indicators that you're ready to advance. Consult with a yoga instructor or observe your ability to maintain proper alignment and engage muscles effectively in more challenging modifications.

Safety and Alignment:

Maintaining Proper Alignment: Focus on aligning your body according to the principles outlined in each modification. Keep your spine elongated, shoulders relaxed, and core engaged. Use props such as blocks or cushions to support proper alignment and prevent strain.

Safety Considerations: Avoid pushing yourself into uncomfortable or painful positions. If you experience discomfort, ease out of the pose, adjust your posture, or switch to a gentler modification. Consult with a healthcare provider or yoga instructor if you have specific concerns about safety.

Incorporating Modifications into Practice:

Mastering Modifications: Start by mastering one modification at a time, focusing on proper alignment and breath awareness. As you become more familiar with each modification, experiment with incorporating different options into your practice session to enhance variety and adaptability.

Transitioning Between Modifications: Transition smoothly between modifications by maintaining mindfulness and breath awareness. Take your time to adjust props or posture as needed to maintain the flow of your chair yoga practice. Practice transitions during slower-paced sessions to build confidence and fluidity.

Personalization of Practice:

Tailoring Modifications: Customize modifications to address specific needs or areas of concern in your body. For example, if you have limited mobility in your hips, modify seated twists by adjusting the degree of rotation or using additional support for the spine.

Additional Resources: Explore resources such as yoga books, online tutorials, or consultations with yoga instructors for more tailored modifications. They can provide personalized guidance based on your individual limitations and goals.

Feedback and Progress Tracking:

Seeking Feedback: It's beneficial to seek feedback from a qualified yoga instructor or healthcare provider to ensure you're using modifications effectively and safely. They can offer adjustments, corrections, and encouragement tailored to your specific needs.
Tracking Progress: Monitor your progress by keeping a journal of your chair yoga practice. Note improvements in flexibility, strength, and overall comfort in using different modifications over time. Celebrate milestones and adjustments that enhance your practice.
Integration with Other Forms of Exercise:

Combining with Other Exercises: Chair yoga modifications can complement other forms of exercise or physical therapy routines. For example, using modified chair yoga poses can enhance flexibility and joint mobility, supporting activities like walking or strength training.
Complementary Modifications: Explore modifications that align with your overall fitness goals and integrate seamlessly into your existing exercise regimen. Consult with healthcare providers or fitness professionals to ensure a balanced approach that supports your overall well-being.
Long-Term Practice Goals:

Setting Realistic Goals: Establish realistic goals for your chair yoga practice, such as improving flexibility, reducing stress, or enhancing relaxation. Use modifications as tools to gradually progress toward these goals while respecting your body's limitations.
Role of Modifications: Modifications play a crucial role in maintaining a consistent chair yoga practice by adapting poses to suit your current abilities and evolving needs. Embrace modifications as a means of promoting sustainable, long-term engagement in yoga for holistic health and well-being.

Chapter 27: Warm-up Exercises for Chair Yoga

Warm-up exercises are essential in chair yoga to prepare the body and mind for the practice ahead. They help increase circulation, improve flexibility, and reduce the risk of injury by gently easing into movement.

1. Neck Rolls
Description: Sit tall with feet flat on the floor. Inhale and slowly drop your chin to your chest. Exhale and roll your head to the right, bringing your ear toward your shoulder. Inhale as you roll your head back to center, then exhale as you roll to the left side. Repeat for several rounds.

Benefits: Relieves tension in the neck and shoulders, improves range of motion in the cervical spine.

2. Shoulder Rolls
Description: Sit tall with arms relaxed by your sides. Inhale as you lift your shoulders up towards your ears. Exhale as you roll them back and down in a smooth, circular motion. Repeat for several rounds, then reverse the direction.

Benefits: Releases tension in the shoulders, improves circulation to the upper body.

3. Seated Cat-Cow Stretch

Description: Sit tall with hands resting on your knees. Inhale as you arch your back, lifting your chest and tilting your pelvis forward (Cow Pose). Exhale as you round your spine, tucking your chin towards your chest (Cat Pose). Flow smoothly between these two positions with your breath.

Benefits: Warms up the spine, stretches the back and abdominal muscles, enhances spinal flexibility.

4. Wrist and Ankle Rotations
Description: Extend your arms forward with palms facing down. Rotate your wrists in circles, first clockwise, then counterclockwise. For ankle rotations, extend one leg forward and rotate your ankle in circles, then switch to the other leg.

Benefits: Increases mobility and flexibility in wrists and ankles, prepares joints for weight-bearing poses.

5. Seated Side Bends
Description: Sit tall with feet flat on the floor. Inhale as you raise one arm overhead, exhale and lean gently to the opposite side. Hold briefly, then inhale back to center and switch sides. Use the chair for support if needed.

Benefits: Stretches the sides of the torso, improves lateral flexibility, prepares for deeper stretches and twists.

6. Gentle Twists
Description: Sit tall with feet flat on the floor. Inhale to lengthen your spine, then exhale and twist gently to one side, placing one hand on the back of the chair and the other on your thigh for support. Hold briefly, then inhale back to center and repeat on the other side.

Benefits: Increases spinal mobility, massages internal organs, improves digestion and detoxification.

Conclusion

These warm-up exercises are designed to prepare your body gradually for chair yoga practice. Start with gentle movements and gradually increase intensity as your body warms up. Incorporating these exercises into your routine will enhance flexibility, circulation, and overall comfort during your chair yoga session. Always listen to your body and modify exercises as needed to suit your individual needs and abilities.

Effectiveness and Purpose:

How do these warm-up exercises specifically benefit chair yoga practice?
Can these warm-ups be adapted for individuals with varying levels of mobility or flexibility?
Integration into Practice:

How many repetitions of each warm-up exercise should I perform before starting my chair yoga session?
Should these warm-ups be done sequentially, or can they be mixed and matched based on personal preference?
Safety and Modifications:

Are there modifications for these warm-up exercises if I have limitations or injuries?
What should I do if I experience discomfort during any of these warm-ups?
Time and Duration:

How long should I spend on warm-up exercises before moving into more challenging chair yoga poses?
Is there a recommended timeframe or sequence for integrating these warm-ups into a chair yoga routine?
Long-Term Benefits:

How will regularly practicing these warm-up exercises improve my overall chair yoga practice?
Can these exercises help prevent injuries or improve flexibility over time?
Personalization and Adaptation:

Can I customize these warm-up exercises to focus on specific areas of stiffness or tension in my body?

Are there additional warm-up exercises that can complement or enhance the ones provided in the chapter?
Progression and Advancement:

As I become more familiar with chair yoga, should I adjust these warm-up exercises to reflect my increasing flexibility and strength?
Are there advanced variations of these warm-up exercises that I can incorporate as I progress in my practice?
Instructor Guidance:

Should I consult with a chair yoga instructor to ensure I'm performing these warm-up exercises correctly?
How can I find resources or videos that demonstrate these warm-up exercises in real-time?

Effectiveness and Purpose:

Benefits of Warm-up Exercises: Warm-up exercises for chair yoga serve to increase blood flow to muscles, enhance joint mobility, and mentally prepare for the practice ahead. Each exercise targets specific areas like the spine, shoulders, and hips, promoting flexibility and reducing the risk of injury during yoga poses.
Adaptability: Yes, these warm-up exercises can be adapted for individuals with varying mobility or flexibility levels. Beginners can start with smaller movements and gradually increase range of motion. For those with limited mobility, modifications such as using props for support or reducing the intensity of stretches can be applied.
Integration into Practice:

Repetition and Sequence: Perform each warm-up exercise 5-10 times, focusing on smooth, controlled movements. Sequentially performing these exercises helps systematically warm up different muscle groups and joints. However, feel free to mix and match based on personal preference or specific needs on any given day.
Safety and Modifications:

Modifications: Modify warm-up exercises by adjusting range of motion or using props (like cushions or straps) to accommodate limitations or injuries. If discomfort arises, reduce the intensity or stop the exercise. Always prioritize comfort and listen to your body's signals to prevent overexertion.
Time and Duration:

Duration: Spend 5-10 minutes on warm-up exercises before progressing to more challenging chair yoga poses. Adjust the duration based on how your body responds and your personal comfort level. Gradually increase the time as your flexibility and stamina improve.
Long-Term Benefits:

Improvement in Practice: Regular practice of these warm-up exercises enhances flexibility, joint mobility, and overall comfort during chair yoga sessions. Over time, they contribute to improved posture, reduced stiffness, and enhanced circulation, which can help prevent injuries and support a deeper yoga practice.
Personalization and Adaptation:

Customization: Customize warm-up exercises to target specific areas of stiffness or tension in your body. For example, if you have tight shoulders, focus on shoulder rolls and gentle twists to release tension. Experiment with additional warm-up exercises or variations recommended by a yoga instructor to tailor your routine to your unique needs.
Progression and Advancement:

Adjusting Exercises: As you advance in chair yoga, adjust warm-up exercises to reflect increased flexibility and strength. Gradually deepen stretches or incorporate more challenging variations (like adding resistance bands or increasing range of motion) to continually progress in your practice.
Instructor Guidance:

Consulting with an Instructor: It's beneficial to consult with a chair yoga instructor to ensure proper alignment and technique in warm-up exercises. They can provide personalized guidance, correct any improper form, and recommend modifications tailored to your specific abilities and goals. Utilize online resources, videos, or local classes to find instructors who specialize in chair yoga for comprehensive guidance.

Chapter 28: Gentle Stretches and Movements to Prepare the Body

In chair yoga, gentle stretches and movements are crucial for warming up muscles, increasing circulation, and enhancing flexibility. These preparatory exercises help to relax the mind and body, promoting a more effective and enjoyable yoga practice.

1. Seated Forward Fold
Description: Sit tall with feet flat on the floor. Inhale to lengthen your spine, then exhale as you hinge at your hips and fold forward, reaching towards your feet or ankles. Hold briefly, feeling a gentle stretch along your spine and the back of your legs. Inhale to rise back up.

Benefits: Stretches the hamstrings, improves flexibility in the spine, and encourages relaxation.

2. Seated Side Stretch
Description: Sit tall with feet flat on the floor. Inhale and reach one arm overhead, exhale and lean gently to the opposite side, keeping the opposite hip grounded. Hold briefly, feeling a stretch along the side of your torso. Inhale back to center and repeat on the other side.

Benefits: Stretches the sides of the body, improves lateral flexibility, and opens the rib cage for deeper breathing.

3. Seated Twist

Description: Sit tall with feet flat on the floor. Inhale to lengthen your spine, then exhale as you twist gently to one side, placing one hand on the back of the chair and the other on your thigh. Hold the twist for a few breaths, feeling a gentle rotation through the spine. Inhale back to center and repeat on the other side.

Benefits: Increases spinal mobility, massages internal organs, and aids in digestion and detoxification.

4. Ankle Rolls
Description: Extend one leg forward, keeping the foot relaxed. Rotate the ankle in circles, first clockwise and then counterclockwise. Switch legs and repeat.

Benefits: Improves mobility in the ankles, enhances circulation in the lower legs, and prepares for weight-bearing poses.

5. Shoulder Shrugs
Description: Sit tall with arms relaxed by your sides. Inhale deeply as you lift your shoulders towards your ears. Exhale and release them down with a gentle sigh. Repeat several times.

Benefits: Relieves tension in the shoulders, increases awareness of shoulder position, and promotes relaxation.

Conclusion
These gentle stretches and movements prepare your body physically and mentally for chair yoga practice. Incorporate them into your warm-up routine to enhance flexibility, circulation, and overall comfort during your yoga session. Listen to your body and modify exercises as needed to suit your individual needs and abilities.

Chapter 29: Chair Yoga Routines

Beginner Routine: Simple Sequence for Those New to Chair Yoga
The beginner routine in chair yoga is designed to introduce foundational poses and gentle movements suitable for individuals who are new to yoga or have limited mobility. This sequence emphasizes comfort, stability, and gradual introduction to the practice.

Routine Overview:
Seated Mountain Pose

Description: Sit tall with feet flat on the floor. Inhale to lengthen your spine, reaching your arms alongside your body with palms facing forward. Hold for a few breaths, focusing on grounding through the feet and lengthening through the spine.
Benefits: Improves posture, enhances awareness of body alignment, and encourages deep breathing.
Seated Cat-Cow Stretch

Description: Sit tall with hands resting on your knees. Inhale as you arch your back, lifting your chest and tilting your pelvis forward (Cow Pose). Exhale as you round your spine, tucking your chin towards your chest (Cat Pose). Flow smoothly between these two positions with your breath.
Benefits: Warms up the spine, stretches the back and abdominal muscles, and improves spinal flexibility.
Chair Forward Fold

Description: Sit tall at the edge of your chair with feet hip-width apart. Inhale to lengthen your spine, then exhale as you hinge forward from your hips, reaching towards your feet or ankles. Hold for a few breaths, feeling a gentle stretch along your spine and the back of your legs.

Benefits: Stretches the hamstrings, relieves tension in the lower back, and promotes relaxation.

Seated Twist

Description: Sit tall with feet flat on the floor. Inhale to lengthen your spine, then exhale as you twist gently to one side, placing one hand on the back of the chair and the other on your thigh. Hold the twist for a few breaths, feeling a gentle rotation through the spine. Inhale back to center and repeat on the other side.

Benefits: Increases spinal mobility, massages internal organs, and aids in digestion.

Seated Side Stretch

Description: Sit tall with feet flat on the floor. Inhale and reach one arm overhead, exhale and lean gently to the opposite side, keeping the opposite hip grounded. Hold briefly, feeling a stretch along the side of your torso. Inhale back to center and repeat on the other side.

Benefits: Stretches the sides of the body, improves lateral flexibility, and enhances breathing capacity.

Conclusion

The beginner chair yoga routine provides a gentle introduction to the practice, focusing on foundational poses that enhance flexibility, posture, and relaxation. Practice these poses regularly to build comfort and confidence in your chair yoga journey. Modify poses as needed to accommodate your body's needs and enjoy the calming benefits of yoga from the comfort of your chair.

Chapter 30: Chair Yoga Routines

Intermediate Routine: More Challenging Poses and Sequences
The intermediate chair yoga routine builds upon the
foundational poses introduced in the beginner routine. It
introduces more challenging poses and sequences to further
enhance strength, flexibility, and mindfulness.

Routine Overview:
Seated Warrior I

Description: Sit tall with feet flat on the floor. Inhale to lift
your arms overhead, palms facing each other. Exhale as you
bend your right knee, keeping the left leg extended and
grounded. Hold the pose for a few breaths, feeling a stretch in
the arms, shoulders, and legs. Repeat on the other side.

Benefits: Strengthens the legs, improves balance, and enhances
concentration.

Chair Crescent Moon

Description: Sit tall with feet flat on the floor. Inhale as you
interlace your fingers and extend your arms overhead, palms
facing upward. Lean gently to the right, feeling a stretch along
the left side of your body. Hold for a few breaths, then inhale
back to center and repeat on the left side.

Benefits: Increases lateral flexibility, stretches the side body,
and promotes relaxation.

Seated Eagle Arms

Description: Sit tall with feet flat on the floor. Inhale to extend your arms straight in front of you at shoulder height. Exhale as you cross your right arm over the left, wrapping the forearms and pressing the palms together. Lift the elbows slightly and hold for a few breaths. Repeat with the left arm over the right.

Benefits: Improves shoulder mobility, releases tension in the upper back and shoulders, and enhances focus.

Seated Twist with Leg Extension

Description: Sit tall with feet flat on the floor. Inhale to lengthen your spine, then exhale as you twist gently to one side, placing one hand on the back of the chair and the other on your thigh. Extend the opposite leg forward, flexing the foot. Hold the twist for a few breaths, feeling a gentle rotation through the spine. Inhale back to center and repeat on the other side.

Benefits: Increases spinal mobility, strengthens the core muscles, and improves circulation.

Seated Pigeon Pose

Description: Sit tall with feet flat on the floor. Cross your right ankle over your left thigh, flexing the right foot. Inhale to lengthen your spine, then exhale as you hinge forward from your hips, keeping the back straight. Hold for a few breaths, feeling a stretch in the outer hip and buttock. Repeat on the other side.

Benefits: Opens the hips, stretches the glutes, and improves flexibility in the hip joints.

Conclusion

The intermediate chair yoga routine challenges your body and mind with more complex poses and sequences. Practice regularly to build strength, flexibility, and mindfulness. Modify poses as needed to accommodate your body's needs and enjoy the transformative benefits of chair yoga.

Chapter 31: Chair Yoga Routines

Advanced Routine: Advanced Chair Yoga Poses for Experienced Practitioners
The advanced chair yoga routine is designed for experienced practitioners looking to deepen their practice with challenging poses that incorporate balance and strength-building exercises.

Routine Overview:
Chair Warrior III

Description: Sit tall at the edge of your chair with feet hip-width apart. Inhale to lift your right leg straight behind you, keeping toes pointing down. Extend your arms forward at shoulder height, palms facing each other. Hold for a few breaths, engaging your core and maintaining a steady gaze.

Benefits: Improves balance, strengthens the legs and core, and enhances concentration and focus.

Seated Tree Pose

Description: Sit tall with feet flat on the floor. Inhale to lift your right foot, placing the sole against your inner left thigh or calf. Bring your palms together at your heart center (Namaste position) or extend your arms overhead. Hold for a few breaths, maintaining balance and alignment. Repeat on the other side.

Benefits: Enhances balance, strengthens the ankles and legs, and promotes mindfulness and poise.

Seated Boat Pose

Description: Sit tall with feet flat on the floor. Inhale as you lift your legs off the floor, balancing on your sitting bones. Extend your arms forward at shoulder height, parallel to the floor. Hold for a few breaths, engaging your core muscles and keeping your spine straight.

Benefits: Strengthens the core muscles, improves balance and stability, and builds abdominal strength.

Chair Dancer's Pose

Description: Sit tall with feet flat on the floor. Inhale to lift your right foot, bringing the heel towards your buttock. Reach your right hand back to hold the ankle or foot, extending your left arm overhead. Hold for a few breaths, gently pressing the foot into the hand to deepen the stretch. Repeat on the other side.

Benefits: Increases flexibility in the quadriceps and hip flexors, enhances balance, and improves posture.

Seated Warrior II

Description: Sit tall with feet wide apart. Inhale to extend your arms out to the sides at shoulder height, palms facing down. Exhale as you bend your right knee, aligning it over the ankle. Gaze over your right fingertips. Hold for a few breaths, feeling a stretch in the legs and opening through the hips. Repeat on the other side.

Benefits: Strengthens the legs and arms, improves stamina and endurance, and cultivates mental resilience.

Conclusion

The advanced chair yoga routine challenges experienced practitioners with complex poses that integrate balance, strength-building, and mindfulness. Practice regularly to refine your skills, deepen your practice, and experience the transformative benefits of advanced chair yoga.

Chapter 32: Specialized Routines

Routines for Specific Needs and Relaxation
This chapter explores specialized chair yoga routines tailored
for specific health concerns such as arthritis, back pain, and
relaxation for stress relief.

1. Arthritis Relief Routine
Description: This routine focuses on gentle movements and
poses that help alleviate joint pain and stiffness associated
with arthritis. Poses include gentle stretches for flexibility and
mobility enhancement, as well as breathing exercises to
promote relaxation.

Benefits: Reduces joint pain and inflammation, improves joint
flexibility and range of motion, and enhances overall well-
being.

2. Back Pain Relief Routine
Description: Designed to relieve tension and discomfort in the
back, this routine includes gentle stretches and strengthening
exercises for the back muscles. Poses emphasize proper
alignment and support to alleviate back pain and improve
spinal health.

Benefits: Strengthens the muscles supporting the spine,
improves posture, reduces back pain and stiffness, and
promotes relaxation.

3. Yoga for Relaxation and Stress Relief

Description: This routine incorporates calming breathing techniques, gentle stretches, and mindfulness practices to reduce stress and promote relaxation. Poses focus on releasing tension from the body and calming the mind, fostering a sense of tranquility and inner peace.

Benefits: Reduces stress and anxiety, improves mental clarity and focus, promotes deep relaxation, and enhances overall emotional well-being.

Conclusion

Specialized chair yoga routines cater to specific health needs and goals, offering tailored practices that promote healing, relaxation, and overall well-being. Practice these routines regularly to experience the therapeutic benefits of chair yoga for your specific concerns.

Chapter 33: Yoga for Specific Health Concerns

Arthritis and Joint Pain
This chapter explores chair yoga poses and routines specifically designed to alleviate symptoms associated with arthritis and joint pain.

Poses and Routines to Alleviate Symptoms:
Gentle Warm-Up

Description: Begin with gentle movements to warm up the joints, such as wrist circles, ankle rotations, and gentle neck stretches. This helps increase circulation and prepare the body for yoga poses.

Benefits: Reduces stiffness, improves joint mobility, and prepares the body for deeper stretches.

Seated Cat-Cow Stretch

Description: Sit tall with hands resting on your knees. Inhale as you arch your back, lifting your chest and tilting your pelvis forward (Cow Pose). Exhale as you round your spine, tucking your chin towards your chest (Cat Pose). Flow smoothly between these two positions with your breath.

Benefits: Increases flexibility in the spine, massages the abdominal organs, and improves posture.

Chair Hip Opener

Description: Sit towards the front edge of your chair with feet flat on the floor. Cross your right ankle over your left thigh, flexing the right foot. Lean forward slightly to deepen the stretch in the outer hip and buttock. Hold for a few breaths, then switch sides.

Benefits: Relieves tension in the hips, improves hip flexibility, and reduces discomfort in the lower back.

Seated Twist

Description: Sit tall with feet flat on the floor. Inhale to lengthen your spine, then exhale as you twist gently to one side, placing one hand on the back of the chair and the other on your thigh. Hold the twist for a few breaths, feeling a gentle rotation through the spine. Inhale back to center and repeat on the other side.

Benefits: Increases spinal mobility, massages internal organs, and improves digestion.

Relaxation Pose

Description: Sit comfortably in your chair with feet flat on the floor. Close your eyes and focus on your breath. Allow your body to relax completely, releasing any tension or stress. Stay in this pose for several minutes, practicing deep breathing and mindful relaxation.

Benefits: Promotes relaxation, reduces stress and anxiety, and supports overall well-being.

Conclusion

Yoga can be a beneficial practice for managing arthritis and joint pain, offering gentle movements and stretches that improve flexibility, reduce stiffness, and promote overall joint health. Incorporate these poses and routines into your daily routine to experience relief and improve your quality of life.

Chapter 34: Yoga for Specific Health Concerns

Back Pain: Strengthening and Stretching Exercises for the Back
This chapter explores chair yoga exercises specifically designed to strengthen and stretch the back, helping to alleviate and prevent back pain.

Strengthening and Stretching Exercises:
Seated Cat-Cow Stretch

Description: Sit tall with hands resting on your knees. Inhale as you arch your back, lifting your chest and tilting your pelvis forward (Cow Pose). Exhale as you round your spine, tucking your chin towards your chest (Cat Pose). Flow smoothly between these two positions with your breath.

Benefits: Increases flexibility in the spine, massages the abdominal organs, and improves posture.

Chair Forward Fold

Description: Sit tall at the edge of your chair with feet hip-width apart. Inhale to lengthen your spine, then exhale as you hinge forward from your hips, reaching towards your feet or ankles. Hold for a few breaths, feeling a gentle stretch along your spine and the back of your legs.

Benefits: Stretches the hamstrings, relieves tension in the lower back, and promotes relaxation.

Seated Twist with Side Bend

Description: Sit tall with feet flat on the floor. Inhale to lengthen your spine, then exhale as you twist gently to one side, placing one hand on the back of the chair and the other on your thigh. Extend the opposite arm overhead, reaching towards the side. Hold for a few breaths, feeling a stretch along the spine and side body. Inhale back to center and repeat on the other side.

Benefits: Increases spinal mobility, stretches the muscles along the spine, and relieves tension in the back.

Chair Bridge Pose

Description: Sit towards the front edge of your chair with feet flat on the floor. Place your hands on the sides of the chair seat, fingers pointing towards your feet. Inhale as you press into your hands and feet, lifting your hips towards the ceiling. Hold for a few breaths, engaging your glutes and core muscles. Exhale to lower back down with control.

Benefits: Strengthens the lower back, glutes, and hamstrings, improves spinal mobility, and relieves back pain.

Seated Locust Pose

Description: Sit tall with feet flat on the floor. Extend your arms straight behind you, palms facing down. Inhale as you lift your chest and legs off the chair, balancing on your sitting bones. Hold for a few breaths, engaging your back muscles. Exhale to release back down with control.

Benefits: Strengthens the muscles along the spine, improves posture, and alleviates tension in the back.

Conclusion

Chair yoga provides effective exercises to strengthen and stretch the back muscles, promoting spine health and alleviating back pain. Incorporate these exercises into your daily routine to build strength, flexibility, and resilience in your back.

Chapter 35: Yoga for Specific Health Concerns

Cardiovascular Health: Yoga Poses to Support Heart Health
This chapter explores chair yoga poses and exercises specifically designed to support cardiovascular health and promote heart health.

Yoga Poses to Support Heart Health:
Seated Mountain Pose

Description: Sit tall with feet flat on the floor, hip-width apart. Place your hands on your knees or thighs, palms facing down. Inhale deeply and lift your chest, lengthening your spine. Hold for a few breaths, focusing on grounding through your sit bones and maintaining steady breathing.

Benefits: Improves posture, enhances circulation, and promotes a sense of grounding and stability.

Chair Warrior II Pose

Description: Sit towards the front edge of your chair with feet wide apart. Inhale to extend your arms out to the sides at shoulder height, palms facing down. Exhale as you bend your right knee, aligning it over the ankle. Gaze over your right fingertips. Hold for a few breaths, feeling a stretch in the legs and opening through the hips. Repeat on the other side.

Benefits: Strengthens the legs and arms, improves stamina and endurance, and supports cardiovascular health.

Seated Forward Fold

Description: Sit tall at the edge of your chair with feet hip-width apart. Inhale to lengthen your spine, then exhale as you hinge forward from your hips, reaching towards your feet or ankles. Hold for a few breaths, feeling a gentle stretch along your spine and the back of your legs.

Benefits: Stretches the hamstrings, improves circulation, and promotes relaxation.

Chair Cat-Cow Stretch

Description: Sit tall with hands resting on your knees. Inhale as you arch your back, lifting your chest and tilting your pelvis forward (Cow Pose). Exhale as you round your spine, tucking your chin towards your chest (Cat Pose). Flow smoothly between these two positions with your breath.

Benefits: Increases flexibility in the spine, massages the abdominal organs, and supports heart health by improving circulation.

Seated Twist

Description: Sit tall with feet flat on the floor. Inhale to lengthen your spine, then exhale as you twist gently to one side, placing one hand on the back of the chair and the other on your thigh. Hold the twist for a few breaths, feeling a gentle rotation through the spine. Inhale back to center and repeat on the other side.

Benefits: Enhances spinal mobility, massages internal organs, and promotes detoxification, supporting overall cardiovascular health.

Conclusion
Chair yoga poses can be beneficial for supporting cardiovascular health by improving circulation, enhancing stamina, and promoting relaxation. Practice these poses regularly to support heart health and overall well-being.

Chapter 36: Yoga for Specific Health Concerns

Osteoporosis: Safe Practices to Maintain Bone Density
This chapter explores safe chair yoga practices designed to help maintain bone density and support overall bone health, especially for individuals with osteoporosis.

Safe Practices to Maintain Bone Density:
Seated Spinal Twist

Description: Sit tall with feet flat on the floor. Inhale to lengthen your spine, then exhale as you twist gently to one side, placing one hand on the back of the chair and the other on your thigh. Hold the twist for a few breaths, feeling a gentle rotation through the spine. Inhale back to center and repeat on the other side.

Benefits: Enhances spinal mobility, stimulates the vertebrae, and supports bone health in the spine.

Seated Side Stretch

Description: Sit tall with feet flat on the floor. Inhale to reach your arms overhead, clasping your hands together. Exhale as you lean gently to one side, lengthening through the spine. Hold for a few breaths, feeling a stretch along the side body. Inhale back to center and repeat on the other side.

Benefits: Stretches the muscles along the sides of the body, improves flexibility, and supports bone health in the ribs and spine.

Chair Warrior I Pose

Description: Sit towards the front edge of your chair with feet hip-width apart. Inhale to extend your arms overhead, palms facing each other. Exhale as you bend your right knee, bringing it over the ankle. Square your hips forward and lift your chest. Hold for a few breaths, feeling a stretch in the front of the left thigh and hip.

Benefits: Strengthens the legs, improves balance, and supports bone health in the legs and hips.

Seated Forward Fold

Description: Sit tall at the edge of your chair with feet hip-width apart. Inhale to lengthen your spine, then exhale as you hinge forward from your hips, reaching towards your feet or ankles. Hold for a few breaths, feeling a gentle stretch along your spine and the back of your legs.

Benefits: Stretches the hamstrings, supports flexibility, and promotes bone health in the spine and legs.

Chair Squat Pose

Description: Stand behind your chair with feet hip-width apart. Inhale as you bend your knees and lower your hips towards the chair, as if sitting down. Keep your chest lifted and knees aligned over the ankles. Hold for a few breaths, then exhale to rise back up.

Benefits: Strengthens the legs, hips, and lower back, supporting bone density in the lower body.

Conclusion
Chair yoga can be a safe and effective practice for individuals with osteoporosis, helping to maintain bone density, improve flexibility, and support overall bone health. Practice these safe poses regularly to enhance bone strength and reduce the risk of fractures.

Chapter 37: Yoga for Specific Health Concerns

Diabetes: Managing Blood Sugar Levels Through Yoga
This chapter explores chair yoga practices specifically designed to help manage blood sugar levels and support overall health for individuals with diabetes.

Managing Blood Sugar Levels Through Yoga:
Seated Forward Fold with Breath Awareness

Description: Sit tall at the edge of your chair with feet hip-width apart. Inhale deeply and extend your arms overhead. Exhale as you hinge forward from your hips, reaching towards your feet or ankles. Hold for a few breaths, focusing on deep abdominal breathing and relaxation.

Benefits: Stimulates digestion, reduces stress, and supports blood sugar regulation.

Seated Spinal Twist

Description: Sit tall with feet flat on the floor. Inhale to lengthen your spine, then exhale as you twist gently to one side, placing one hand on the back of the chair and the other on your thigh. Hold the twist for a few breaths, feeling a gentle rotation through the spine. Inhale back to center and repeat on the other side.

Benefits: Improves digestion, massages internal organs, and supports insulin sensitivity.

Chair Cat-Cow Stretch

Description: Sit tall with hands resting on your knees. Inhale as you arch your back, lifting your chest and tilting your pelvis forward (Cow Pose). Exhale as you round your spine, tucking your chin towards your chest (Cat Pose). Flow smoothly between these two positions with your breath.

Benefits: Enhances spinal flexibility, stimulates the abdominal organs, and supports digestion and blood sugar regulation.

Chair Warrior II Pose

Description: Sit towards the front edge of your chair with feet wide apart. Inhale to extend your arms out to the sides at shoulder height, palms facing down. Exhale as you bend your right knee, aligning it over the ankle. Gaze over your right fingertips. Hold for a few breaths, feeling a stretch in the legs and opening through the hips. Repeat on the other side.

Benefits: Strengthens the legs, improves circulation, and supports overall metabolic health.

Seated Relaxation Pose

Description: Sit comfortably in your chair with feet flat on the floor. Close your eyes and focus on your breath. Allow your body to relax completely, releasing any tension or stress. Stay in this pose for several minutes, practicing deep breathing and mindful relaxation.

Benefits: Reduces stress and anxiety, supports overall well-being, and helps regulate blood sugar levels.

Conclusion
Chair yoga can be a valuable tool for managing diabetes by promoting relaxation, improving circulation, and supporting overall health. Practice these yoga poses regularly to help maintain stable blood sugar levels and enhance your well-being.

Chapter 38: Enhancing Your Practice

Incorporating Mindfulness: Techniques for Mindfulness and Meditation
This chapter explores techniques for integrating mindfulness and meditation into chair yoga practice to enhance overall well-being.

Techniques for Mindfulness and Meditation:
Mindful Breathing

Description: Sit comfortably in your chair with feet flat on the floor and hands resting on your thighs. Close your eyes or gaze softly downwards. Begin to observe your breath without trying to change it. Notice the sensations of the breath as it enters and leaves your body. If your mind wanders, gently bring your focus back to your breath.

Benefits: Calms the mind, reduces stress and anxiety, enhances focus, and promotes relaxation.

Body Scan Meditation

Description: Sit comfortably and close your eyes. Begin to bring awareness to different parts of your body, starting from the top of your head down to your toes. Notice any sensations, tension, or relaxation in each part. Breathe into areas of tension and visualize them releasing with each exhale.

Benefits: Promotes relaxation, increases body awareness, and helps release tension and stress.

Guided Visualization

Description: Sit comfortably and close your eyes. Visualize a peaceful and relaxing place, such as a beach or a serene garden. Imagine yourself there, noticing the sights, sounds, and smells. Engage all your senses in this visualization, allowing yourself to fully immerse in the experience.

Benefits: Reduces stress and anxiety, enhances relaxation, and improves mood and overall well-being.

Mantra Meditation

Description: Choose a word, phrase, or sound (mantra) that resonates with you. Sit comfortably and silently repeat the mantra to yourself with each inhale and exhale. Allow the mantra to anchor your mind and bring your focus inward.

Benefits: Calms the mind, promotes concentration, and enhances mindfulness and self-awareness.

Mindful Movement

Description: Practice yoga poses with mindfulness, focusing on each movement and breath. Notice how your body feels in each pose, and observe any thoughts or sensations that arise without judgment. Stay present and connected to the experience of practicing chair yoga.

Benefits: Enhances body awareness, improves concentration, and deepens the connection between mind and body.

Conclusion

Incorporating mindfulness and meditation techniques into chair yoga practice can enrich your experience, promote relaxation, and support overall well-being. Explore these techniques regularly to cultivate mindfulness, reduce stress, and enhance your practice.

Chapter 39: Nutrition and Hydration

Importance of Diet and Hydration for Yoga Practice
This chapter explores the significance of maintaining a
balanced diet and adequate hydration to support optimal
performance and well-being during chair yoga practice.

Importance of Diet:
Balanced Nutrition

Description: Emphasize a diet rich in fruits, vegetables, whole
grains, lean proteins, and healthy fats. Incorporate foods that
provide sustained energy and support muscle recovery.

Benefits: Provides essential nutrients for overall health,
supports muscle function and repair, and enhances energy
levels during yoga practice.

Timing of Meals

Description: Plan meals and snacks to fuel your body
adequately before and after chair yoga sessions. Avoid heavy
meals that may cause discomfort during practice.

Benefits: Maintains stable blood sugar levels, supports
digestion, and optimizes energy levels for yoga practice.

Hydration

Description: Drink water throughout the day to stay hydrated.
Aim to drink water before, during, and after chair yoga
practice to replenish fluids lost through sweating.

Benefits: Supports joint lubrication, regulates body temperature, enhances mental clarity, and improves overall performance during yoga practice.

Importance of Hydration:
Hydration Guidelines

Description: Consume adequate water based on your individual needs and activity level. Monitor hydration by paying attention to thirst cues and the color of your urine (pale yellow indicates adequate hydration).

Benefits: Prevents dehydration, supports cardiovascular health, improves circulation, and aids in detoxification.

Electrolyte Balance

Description: Include electrolyte-rich foods and beverages (such as coconut water or sports drinks) if practicing chair yoga in a warm environment or for prolonged periods to replenish electrolytes lost through sweat.

Benefits: Maintains fluid balance, supports muscle function, and enhances overall hydration status.

Conclusion
Maintaining a balanced diet and adequate hydration is crucial for supporting optimal performance, energy levels, and overall well-being during chair yoga practice. Prioritize nutritious foods and hydration to enhance your yoga experience and promote long-term health.

Chapter 40: Maintaining Consistency

Tips for Staying Motivated and Making Yoga a Habit
This chapter explores strategies and tips to help individuals stay motivated and establish a consistent chair yoga practice as a regular habit.

Tips for Staying Motivated:
Set Realistic Goals

Description: Establish achievable goals for your chair yoga practice, such as practicing a certain number of times per week or mastering specific poses. Break larger goals into smaller milestones to track progress.

Benefits: Provides clarity and motivation, boosts confidence, and fosters a sense of accomplishment.

Create a Routine

Description: Designate specific times and days for chair yoga practice that fit into your daily schedule. Establishing a routine helps to make yoga a regular part of your lifestyle.

Benefits: Builds consistency, reinforces habit formation, and minimizes decision-making.

Find Enjoyment

Description: Explore different chair yoga routines and styles to find what resonates with you. Choose practices that you enjoy and look forward to, whether it's gentle stretching, relaxation techniques, or more challenging sequences.

Benefits: Enhances motivation, fosters a positive attitude towards practice, and increases overall satisfaction.

Making Yoga a Habit:
Start Small

Description: Begin with shorter chair yoga sessions if establishing a regular practice is challenging. Even a few minutes of practice can be beneficial. Gradually increase the duration and intensity as your consistency improves.

Benefits: Reduces barriers to starting, builds momentum, and establishes a foundation for long-term commitment.

Create a Supportive Environment

Description: Surround yourself with supportive resources and individuals who encourage your yoga practice. Join a chair yoga class or community, engage with online forums or social media groups, or practice with a friend or family member.

Benefits: Provides accountability, encouragement, and a sense of community, which can enhance motivation and commitment.

Track Your Progress

Description: Keep a yoga journal or use a tracking app to monitor your practice sessions, progress in poses, and how you feel before and after practice. Celebrate milestones and reflect on your journey.

Benefits: Provides visual feedback of your efforts, boosts motivation, and reinforces the habit of consistent practice.

Conclusion
Establishing a consistent chair yoga practice requires dedication and effort, but it can significantly enhance your physical, mental, and emotional well-being. Incorporate these tips into your routine to stay motivated, build consistency, and reap the benefits of a regular yoga practice.

Chapter 41: Community and Support

Finding a Class: How to Choose a Chair Yoga Class
This chapter explores considerations and tips for finding a suitable chair yoga class that meets your needs and supports your practice.

How to Choose a Chair Yoga Class:
Location and Accessibility

Description: Consider the location of the class and how accessible it is for you. Choose a class that is conveniently located and easy to access, whether it's near your home, workplace, or community center.

Benefits: Reduces barriers to attendance, enhances convenience, and supports regular participation.

Instructor Qualifications

Description: Research the qualifications and experience of the chair yoga instructor. Look for instructors who are certified in teaching yoga to seniors or individuals with specific health concerns. Consider their background in chair yoga and their ability to modify poses for different abilities.

Benefits: Ensures safe and effective instruction, provides expertise in adapting yoga for seniors, and promotes confidence in the instructor's knowledge.

Class Format and Focus

Description: Evaluate the class format and structure. Determine if the class focuses on gentle stretching, relaxation techniques, strength-building exercises, or a combination of these elements. Choose a class that aligns with your goals and preferences.

Benefits: Tailors the practice to your specific needs, enhances engagement, and supports your desired outcomes from chair yoga.

Class Atmosphere and Environment

Description: Visit the class or speak with current participants to get a sense of the atmosphere and environment. Assess if the class environment is welcoming, supportive, and inclusive. Consider factors such as class size, ambiance, and the overall vibe.

Benefits: Creates a positive experience, fosters community and connection, and enhances enjoyment and motivation.

Trial Classes and Feedback

Description: Attend trial classes or introductory sessions if available. Use this opportunity to experience the class firsthand, interact with the instructor, and assess how comfortable you feel with the class format and teaching style. Seek feedback from participants to gain insights into their experiences.

Benefits: Allows for informed decision-making, ensures compatibility with your preferences, and promotes confidence in your choice of chair yoga class.

Conclusion
Choosing a chair yoga class that suits your needs and preferences is essential for enjoying a positive and beneficial yoga experience. Consider these factors when selecting a class to support your journey towards improved health and well-being through chair yoga practice.

Chapter 42: Benefits of Practicing with a Group

Support Networks and Communities
This chapter explores the advantages of participating in chair yoga classes within a supportive group environment and the benefits of community engagement.

Benefits of Practicing with a Group:
Motivation and Accountability

Description: Practicing chair yoga in a group setting provides motivation and accountability. Sharing the experience with others encourages regular attendance and commitment to your practice.

Benefits: Enhances consistency, boosts motivation, and promotes adherence to your chair yoga routine.

Social Connection

Description: Engaging in chair yoga classes allows you to connect with like-minded individuals who share an interest in health and well-being. Building friendships and social connections within the group can reduce feelings of isolation and loneliness.

Benefits: Fosters a sense of belonging, enhances social support, and promotes overall mental and emotional well-being.

Skill Development and Learning

Description: Practicing chair yoga in a group setting offers opportunities for skill development and learning. Observing others and receiving guidance from the instructor can deepen your understanding of poses and techniques.

Benefits: Accelerates learning, improves technique, and provides feedback and encouragement from peers and the instructor.

Sense of Community

Description: Being part of a chair yoga class creates a sense of community and shared purpose. Celebrating achievements, supporting each other through challenges, and sharing experiences create a supportive and uplifting atmosphere.

Benefits: Cultivates empathy, compassion, and camaraderie, enhancing the overall enjoyment and satisfaction of your chair yoga practice.

Emotional Support and Encouragement

Description: Group settings provide emotional support and encouragement during chair yoga practice. Sharing successes, discussing challenges, and receiving encouragement from others can boost confidence and resilience.

Benefits: Provides emotional resilience, promotes positive self-esteem, and enhances the enjoyment of chair yoga practice.

Conclusion

Participating in chair yoga classes within a supportive group environment offers numerous benefits for physical, mental, and emotional well-being. Embrace the opportunity to engage with a community of peers who share your passion for health and wellness through chair yoga practice.

Chapter 43: Frequently Asked Questions

Common Concerns: Addressing Fears and Misconceptions about Chair Yoga
This chapter addresses common concerns, fears, and misconceptions that individuals may have about practicing chair yoga, providing clarity and guidance.

Addressing Fears and Misconceptions:
Fear of Injury

Concern: Will chair yoga cause injury, especially for seniors or individuals with limited mobility?

Response: Chair yoga is specifically designed to be safe and accessible for individuals of all ages and abilities. Poses can be modified to suit your comfort level, and instructors are trained to provide guidance on proper alignment and technique to prevent injury.

Misconception of Difficulty

Concern: Is chair yoga too easy or not effective compared to traditional yoga?

Response: Chair yoga offers a gentle approach to yoga practice that focuses on flexibility, strength, and relaxation. It can be as challenging or gentle as needed, with poses and routines adapted to individual abilities. The effectiveness of chair yoga lies in its ability to improve physical and mental well-being without the strain of more intense practices.

Perception of Limitations

Concern: Will chair yoga be limiting or less beneficial than other forms of exercise?

Response: Chair yoga is highly beneficial for seniors and individuals with mobility issues or health concerns. It enhances flexibility, strength, balance, and mental clarity while reducing stress. It complements other forms of exercise and can be adapted to suit various health conditions and fitness levels.

Troubleshooting:
Difficulty with Poses

Issue: What should I do if I find certain poses challenging or uncomfortable?

Solution: Communicate with your instructor about any discomfort or difficulty with poses. They can offer modifications or alternative poses to accommodate your needs and ensure a safe and enjoyable practice.

Lack of Progress

Issue: What if I feel like I'm not making progress in my chair yoga practice?

Solution: Progress in yoga is gradual and personal. Focus on the benefits you experience, such as improved flexibility, reduced stress, or enhanced relaxation. Set realistic goals and celebrate small achievements to stay motivated.

Time Commitment

Issue: How can I fit chair yoga into my busy schedule?

Solution: Incorporate chair yoga into your daily routine by scheduling short practice sessions. Even a few minutes of practice can provide benefits. Consider attending group classes for accountability and motivation or practicing at home using resources like online videos or apps.

Conclusion
Addressing common concerns, fears, and misconceptions about chair yoga empowers individuals to embrace this gentle and effective form of exercise. By troubleshooting challenges and providing clarity, chair yoga becomes accessible and enjoyable, promoting overall health and well-being.

Chapter 44: Solutions to Common Issues and Progressing Safely

Solutions to Common Issues (e.g., discomfort, difficulty with poses)
This chapter addresses common challenges individuals may face during chair yoga practice and provides practical solutions to ensure a safe and enjoyable experience.

Solutions to Common Issues:
Discomfort during Poses

Issue: What should I do if I experience discomfort or strain during chair yoga poses?

Solution: Listen to your body and modify or skip poses that cause discomfort. Communicate with your instructor about any concerns and ask for alternative poses or adjustments to improve comfort and safety.

Difficulty with Balance

Issue: How can I improve balance during chair yoga poses?

Solution: Use the chair for support and stability during balance poses. Start with simpler poses and gradually progress to more challenging variations as your balance improves. Focus on engaging core muscles and maintaining a steady breath.

Flexibility Challenges

Issue: What if I have limited flexibility? How can I adapt poses to my abilities?

Solution: Modify poses by using props like yoga blocks or straps to support and extend your reach. Incorporate gentle stretching and warm-up exercises before practice to increase flexibility gradually over time.

Breathing Difficulties

Issue: How can I improve my breathing techniques during chair yoga?

Solution: Practice mindful breathing techniques such as deep belly breathing or paced breathing exercises. Focus on inhaling and exhaling slowly and steadily, coordinating breath with movement to enhance relaxation and concentration.

Progressing Safely:
Gradual Progression

Strategy: Start with beginner-level poses and routines, focusing on mastering foundational techniques and building confidence. Gradually progress to intermediate and advanced poses as you gain strength, flexibility, and experience.

Benefit: Minimizes the risk of injury, allows for adaptation to individual abilities, and promotes steady improvement in chair yoga practice.

Consultation with Healthcare Provider

Strategy: Before progressing to more challenging poses or routines, consult your healthcare provider, especially if you have underlying health conditions or concerns. Discuss your chair yoga practice and seek advice on safe progression.

Benefit: Ensures personalized guidance, addresses health considerations, and promotes safe and effective chair yoga practice tailored to your needs.

Mindful Practice

Strategy: Practice mindfulness and self-awareness during chair yoga sessions. Listen to your body's signals, respect your limits, and avoid pushing yourself beyond comfortable ranges of motion or exertion.

Benefit: Enhances self-care, promotes mindfulness in movement, and fosters a positive relationship with your yoga practice.

Conclusion
By addressing common issues and focusing on safe progression, individuals can enjoy the benefits of chair yoga while minimizing challenges and maximizing enjoyment and well-being. Incorporate these solutions into your practice to ensure a fulfilling and sustainable chair yoga experience.

Chapter 45: How to Know When to Advance Your Practice

Knowing When to Advance Your Practice
This chapter explores signs, considerations, and strategies for determining when to progress to more advanced levels in chair yoga.

Signs and Considerations:
Comfort and Confidence

Sign: Feeling comfortable and confident in performing basic chair yoga poses and routines without significant discomfort or strain.

Consideration: Assess your readiness to explore more challenging poses and sequences based on your comfort level and ability to maintain proper form and alignment.

Physical Progress

Sign: Noticing improvements in flexibility, strength, and balance as a result of regular chair yoga practice.

Consideration: Recognize physical advancements and consider advancing your practice to incorporate more demanding poses or intensify existing routines to further enhance your capabilities.

Emotional and Mental Awareness

Sign: Experiencing enhanced mindfulness, relaxation, and mental clarity during chair yoga sessions.

Consideration: Pay attention to emotional and mental benefits gained from chair yoga practice. When ready, challenge yourself with more complex sequences or incorporate meditation techniques to deepen your practice.

Strategies for Advancement:
Consultation with Instructor

Strategy: Seek guidance from your chair yoga instructor to assess your readiness for advancement. Discuss your goals, strengths, and areas for improvement to receive personalized recommendations.

Benefit: Receives expert advice, ensures proper progression, and enhances understanding of your practice's potential.

Exploration of New Techniques

Strategy: Explore new chair yoga techniques, poses, or variations to expand your repertoire and challenge yourself.

Benefit: Promotes continuous learning, stimulates growth in practice, and maintains engagement and interest in chair yoga.

Integration of Mind-Body Practices

Strategy: Integrate mindfulness, meditation, or breathing exercises into your chair yoga practice to deepen relaxation and concentration.

Benefit: Cultivates holistic well-being, improves mental focus, and supports overall health benefits from chair yoga.

Conclusion
Advancing your chair yoga practice involves recognizing personal growth, readiness, and commitment to further explore and challenge yourself in a safe and supportive manner. By understanding signs of readiness and employing strategic approaches, you can enhance your chair yoga experience and achieve continued progress and well-being.

Chapter 46: Stories and Testimonials - Real-Life Experiences

Real-Life Experiences
This chapter shares personal stories, testimonials, and experiences of individuals who have benefited from chair yoga, highlighting its impact on their physical, mental, and emotional well-being.

Personal Stories and Testimonials:
Improvements in Mobility and Flexibility

Story: Jane, 68, shares how chair yoga helped her regain flexibility and mobility after knee surgery. She discusses specific poses and routines that contributed to her recovery and enhanced her overall quality of life.

Testimonial: "Chair yoga has been a game-changer for me. I never thought I could regain the flexibility in my knees, but with consistent practice, I can now move with ease and comfort."

Stress Reduction and Mental Clarity

Story: John, 72, talks about his journey with chair yoga to manage stress and improve mental clarity. He describes the breathing techniques and meditation practices that have helped him find peace and focus in his daily life.

Testimonial: "Chair yoga isn't just about physical benefits; it's about finding inner peace. The mindfulness techniques taught in class have transformed how I approach challenges and enjoy each moment."

Community and Support

Story: Sarah, 70, shares her experience of joining a chair yoga group and the sense of community and support it has provided. She discusses the friendships formed and the encouragement received from fellow practitioners.

Testimonial: "Practicing chair yoga with others has been incredibly uplifting. We cheer each other on, share our successes, and motivate one another to keep coming back. It's more than just exercise; it's a supportive community."

Conclusion
The real-life experiences, stories, and testimonials shared in this chapter illustrate the diverse benefits and profound impact of chair yoga on individuals' lives. By hearing these personal journeys, readers can gain inspiration, motivation, and a deeper understanding of how chair yoga can enhance physical health, mental clarity, and emotional resilience.

Glossary: Definitions of Common Yoga Terms and Concepts

This chapter provides definitions and explanations of key yoga terms and concepts frequently used in chair yoga practice.

Yoga Terms and Concepts:
Asana

Definition: A yoga pose or posture designed to promote physical health and mental well-being. In chair yoga, asanas are adapted to be performed while seated or using a chair for support.
Pranayama

Definition: Breath control exercises in yoga aimed at regulating and enhancing the flow of prana (life force energy) through the body. In chair yoga, pranayama techniques can be practiced while seated comfortably.
Meditation

Definition: A practice of focused attention and mindfulness to cultivate inner peace, clarity, and emotional balance. In chair yoga, meditation techniques are adapted to support relaxation and mental clarity.
Mindfulness

Definition: The practice of being present and aware of one's thoughts, feelings, and sensations without judgment. Chair yoga incorporates mindfulness techniques to enhance self-awareness and reduce stress.
Alignment

Definition: The correct positioning of the body in yoga poses to achieve optimal balance, stability, and energy flow. In chair yoga, alignment is essential for safe and effective practice, often guided by instructors.
Props

Definition: Tools such as yoga blocks, straps, bolsters, and blankets used to support and enhance yoga practice. In chair yoga, props are utilized to modify poses and accommodate individual needs.
Chakra

Definition: Energy centers in the subtle body according to yoga philosophy. Each chakra is associated with specific qualities and organs, and chair yoga may include practices to balance and activate these energy centers.
Savasana

Definition: The final relaxation pose practiced at the end of a yoga session to integrate the benefits of yoga practice and promote deep relaxation and rejuvenation. In chair yoga, savasana can be adapted for seated relaxation.
Additional Terms:
Vinyasa: A sequence of poses coordinated with breath.

Namaste: A greeting and gesture of respect often used to conclude a yoga class.

Om: A sacred sound and mantra often chanted at the beginning or end of yoga practice.

Yogi/Yogini: Terms referring to a practitioner of yoga, often used to denote someone who follows the yoga path.

Conclusion

The glossary provides definitions of essential yoga terms and concepts to enhance understanding and deepen appreciation of chair yoga practice. By familiarizing yourself with these terms, you can navigate and enrich your yoga journey with confidence and clarity.

Conclusion: Recap of Benefits

This chapter summarizes the wide-ranging benefits of chair yoga, emphasizing its positive impact on physical health, mental well-being, and overall quality of life.

Recap of Benefits:
Physical Benefits

Flexibility: Chair yoga improves joint mobility and flexibility, making daily movements easier and reducing stiffness.
Strength: Gentle resistance exercises help maintain and build muscle strength, crucial for balance and stability.
Balance: Practice enhances balance and coordination, reducing the risk of falls and injuries.
Mental Benefits

Stress Reduction: Techniques like deep breathing and meditation promote relaxation and alleviate stress.
Mental Clarity: Chair yoga enhances focus, concentration, and cognitive function, improving overall mental well-being.
Emotional Balance: Regular practice fosters emotional resilience and a sense of inner calm.
Emotional and Social Benefits

Community Engagement: Joining chair yoga classes fosters a sense of belonging and social connection, reducing feelings of isolation.

Supportive Environment: Sharing experiences with others encourages mutual support and motivation, enhancing overall well-being.

Key Points to Remember:

Accessibility: Chair yoga is accessible to individuals of all ages and fitness levels, including those with mobility challenges or health concerns.

Adaptability: Poses and routines can be modified to suit individual needs and abilities, ensuring a safe and personalized practice.

Holistic Approach: Integrates physical movement, breath awareness, and mindfulness practices to promote holistic health and wellness.

Encouragement and Motivation:

Continued Practice: Embrace chair yoga as a lifelong practice to sustain health benefits and enhance overall quality of life.

Personal Growth: Celebrate progress and improvements in physical, mental, and emotional well-being through consistent chair yoga practice.

Final Thoughts:

Chair yoga offers a gentle yet effective way to maintain or improve health and vitality at any stage of life. By incorporating chair yoga into your routine, you can experience the profound benefits it brings to your mind, body, and spirit.

Final Thoughts: Encouragement to Embrace a Healthy and Active Lifestyle

This concluding chapter inspires readers to adopt and maintain a healthy, active lifestyle with chair yoga as a cornerstone of their well-being.

Embracing Health and Wellness:
Lifelong Journey

Chair yoga is not just an exercise but a journey towards better health and well-being that can be sustained throughout life.
Holistic Approach

Integrating chair yoga into your daily routine supports overall health, encompassing physical, mental, and emotional aspects.
Consistency and Progress

Consistent practice yields gradual improvements in flexibility, strength, balance, and mental clarity. Celebrate each milestone along the way.
Chair Yoga as a Foundation:

Accessibility: Chair yoga is inclusive and accessible to people of all ages and abilities, offering modifications to suit individual needs.

Mind-Body Connection: Enhance self-awareness, mindfulness, and relaxation through mindful movement and breathwork.

Community Support: Engaging in chair yoga classes fosters a sense of community and support, enhancing motivation and enjoyment.

Embracing a Healthy Lifestyle:
Nutrition and Hydration: Complement chair yoga with a balanced diet and adequate hydration to support overall health.

Physical Activity: Incorporate other forms of physical activity that complement chair yoga, such as walking, swimming, or gentle stretching.

Mindful Living: Apply principles learned in chair yoga—like mindfulness and stress management—to daily life for a more balanced and fulfilling lifestyle.

Moving Forward:
Setting Goals: Establish realistic goals for your chair yoga practice and health journey, focusing on progress and personal growth.

Seeking Support: Connect with healthcare providers and yoga instructors for guidance and support on your wellness journey.

Conclusion:

Chair yoga empowers individuals to take charge of their health and well-being in a gentle yet effective manner. By embracing a healthy and active lifestyle supported by chair yoga, you can cultivate vitality, resilience, and joy in every stage of life.

Appendix A: Health and Safety Checklist

This appendix provides a comprehensive checklist to ensure a safe and effective chair yoga practice environment.

Health and Safety Checklist:
Consultation with Healthcare Provider:

Before starting chair yoga, consult with your healthcare provider to assess any health concerns or conditions that may affect your practice.
Physical Environment:

Choose a quiet and well-ventilated space for practicing chair yoga.
Ensure the area is free from obstacles and hazards that could cause tripping or falling.
Chair Selection:

Select a sturdy chair with a flat seat and backrest that provides ample support.
Avoid chairs with wheels or arms that may hinder movement during practice.
Personal Comfort:

Wear comfortable clothing that allows for ease of movement and does not restrict circulation.
Use a yoga mat or non-slip surface under the chair to prevent it from sliding.
Warm-up and Cool-down:

Begin each session with gentle warm-up exercises to prepare the body for movement.
Conclude each session with relaxation techniques or a cool-down to ease tension and promote relaxation.
Hydration and Nutrition:

Stay hydrated before, during, and after chair yoga practice.
Maintain a balanced diet to support energy levels and overall well-being.
Listening to Your Body:

Practice mindfulness and listen to your body's signals during chair yoga.
Modify poses or take breaks as needed to prevent strain or injury.
Emergency Preparedness:

Keep emergency contact information readily available in case of medical emergencies.
Familiarize yourself with basic first aid procedures and have necessary supplies nearby.
Progression and Adjustment:

Gradually progress in chair yoga practice as you become more comfortable and confident.
Adjust poses and routines based on individual abilities and limitations.
Conclusion:
This health and safety checklist serves as a guide to creating a safe and supportive environment for chair yoga practice. By prioritizing health considerations and following safety protocols, practitioners can enjoy the benefits of chair yoga with confidence and peace of mind.

Ensuring a Safe Practice Environment

Creating a safe environment for chair yoga practice is essential to enhance comfort, prevent injuries, and optimize the benefits of the practice. Here are key considerations to ensure safety:

Physical Environment:
Space and Setup:

Choose a spacious area free of clutter and obstacles to allow for easy movement around the chair.
Ensure adequate lighting and ventilation to maintain a comfortable atmosphere during practice.
Chair Selection:

Select a sturdy chair with a flat seat and backrest that provides sufficient support.

Avoid chairs with wheels or unstable bases that could compromise stability during poses.
Floor Surface:

Place the chair on a non-slip surface or yoga mat to prevent it from sliding during movements.
Ensure the area around the chair is free from rugs or carpets that could cause tripping hazards.
Personal Comfort and Safety:
Clothing:

Wear comfortable, loose-fitting clothing that allows for unrestricted movement.
Avoid clothing with dangling strings or accessories that could get caught in the chair or impede movement.
Footwear:

Practice barefoot or wear non-slip socks to maintain stability and prevent slipping on smooth surfaces.
Avoid shoes that could mark or damage the floor surface.
Accessibility:

Make sure the chair is easily accessible, especially for individuals with mobility limitations or using assistive devices.
Adjust the height of the chair if necessary to ensure a comfortable and stable seated position.
Instructor Guidance and Supervision:
Qualified Instruction:

Practice under the guidance of a qualified chair yoga instructor who understands the specific needs and abilities of seniors.
The instructor should provide clear instructions, modifications for different levels, and ensure proper alignment during poses.

Monitoring Participants:

The instructor should monitor participants closely for signs of discomfort, fatigue, or difficulty with poses.
Encourage open communication between participants and the instructor to address any concerns or adjustments needed.
Emergency Preparedness:
Emergency Contacts:

Keep emergency contact information readily available in case of medical emergencies or unexpected incidents.
Inform participants of the location of emergency exits and procedures for summoning assistance if needed.
First Aid Kit:

Have a well-stocked first aid kit accessible in the practice area, equipped with basic medical supplies and emergency aids.
Ensure the instructor is trained in basic first aid procedures and knows how to respond appropriately in case of injuries.
Conclusion:
By prioritizing these safety considerations, practitioners can create a supportive and secure environment for chair yoga practice. Whether practicing at home or in a group setting, ensuring a safe practice environment enhances the enjoyment and benefits of chair yoga for all participants.

Summary of Key Points for Ensuring a Safe Practice Environment

Physical Environment:

Space and Setup: Choose a spacious, clutter-free area with good lighting and ventilation.
Chair Selection: Use a sturdy chair with a flat seat and backrest for stability and support.
Floor Surface: Place the chair on a non-slip surface or yoga mat to prevent slipping.
Personal Comfort and Safety:

Clothing: Wear comfortable, loose-fitting clothing suitable for movement.
Footwear: Practice barefoot or wear non-slip socks to maintain stability.
Accessibility: Ensure the chair is easily accessible and adjusted for individual comfort.
Instructor Guidance:

Practice under the guidance of a qualified chair yoga instructor.
The instructor should provide clear instructions, modifications, and ensure proper alignment.
Monitoring and Communication:

The instructor should monitor participants for signs of discomfort or fatigue.
Encourage open communication between participants and the instructor.
Emergency Preparedness:

Keep emergency contact information readily available.
Have a first aid kit accessible and ensure the instructor is trained in basic first aid.
Practice Modifications:

Adapt poses and routines to suit individual abilities and limitations.
Focus on gradual progression and avoid pushing beyond comfortable limits.
Participant Awareness:

Participants should listen to their bodies and respect personal limits.
Report any concerns or discomfort to the instructor promptly.
Consistency in Safety Practices:

Maintain consistent safety protocols in every chair yoga session.
Regularly review and update safety measures as needed.
Conclusion
By prioritizing safety considerations in chair yoga practice, participants can enjoy the benefits of yoga in a secure and supportive environment. These key points ensure that each session is both effective and enjoyable, promoting overall well-being and minimizing the risk of injury.

Useful Contacts

Organizations and Groups Related to Senior Fitness and Yoga
SilverSneakers

Website: silversneakers.com
Description: SilverSneakers offers fitness programs for seniors, including yoga classes tailored to older adults' needs. They provide access to gyms and community centers across the United States.
AARP

Website: aarp.org

Description: AARP provides resources and information on health, fitness, and wellness for seniors, including articles and guides on chair yoga and other fitness activities.
National Council on Aging (NCOA)

Website: ncoa.org
Description: NCOA promotes healthy aging through programs and resources focused on fitness, including evidence-based exercise programs like chair yoga for seniors.
Local Community Centers

Contact your local community centers or senior centers for information on chair yoga classes and fitness programs available in your area.
They often host classes specifically designed for seniors and can provide information on schedules, instructors, and accessibility.
Yoga Alliance

Website: yogaalliance.org
Description: Yoga Alliance is a global organization supporting yoga teachers, schools, and practitioners. They offer resources on yoga styles, including chair yoga, and can help locate certified instructors.
Local Yoga Studios

Check with local yoga studios for information on chair yoga classes tailored for seniors. Many studios offer specialized programs and workshops focused on accessible yoga practices.
Conclusion

These organizations and contacts provide valuable resources and support for seniors interested in chair yoga and overall fitness. Whether seeking classes, information, or community engagement, these resources can help individuals maintain health and well-being through yoga and related fitness activities.

Encouragement and Motivation

This final section aims to inspire and motivate seniors to continue their chair yoga practice with enthusiasm and dedication.

Recognizing Progress and Achievements:
Celebrate Milestones:

Acknowledge and celebrate each step forward in your chair yoga journey, whether it's mastering a new pose or experiencing increased flexibility.
Setting Realistic Goals:

Establish achievable goals for your practice, focusing on personal growth and improvement rather than comparison with others.
Embracing Challenges:

Challenges in your practice are opportunities for growth. Embrace them with patience and persistence, knowing that progress takes time.
Embracing a Holistic Approach to Well-being:
Mind-Body Connection:

Cultivate awareness of the mind-body connection through chair yoga. Notice how your physical practice impacts your mental and emotional well-being.
Stress Reduction:

Utilize chair yoga as a tool for stress relief and relaxation. Incorporate deep breathing and mindfulness techniques into your daily routine.
Community and Support:

Engage with fellow practitioners and support networks to share experiences and encourage each other's journey in chair yoga.
Long-term Benefits and Commitment:
Health Benefits:

Reflect on the physical, mental, and emotional benefits you've experienced through chair yoga. Use these insights to maintain motivation.
Consistency and Routine:

Establish a consistent chair yoga practice schedule that fits into your daily life. Consistency fosters progress and enhances overall well-being.

Gratitude and Mindfulness:

Practice gratitude for the opportunity to engage in chair yoga and enhance your quality of life. Approach each practice with mindfulness and intention.

Conclusion:

Chair yoga offers seniors a gentle yet powerful way to nurture their health and vitality. By staying committed, setting goals, and embracing the journey with positivity, you can continue to reap the benefits of chair yoga for years to come.

Appendix B: Weekly Practice Planner

Use this template to plan and organize your chair yoga sessions throughout the week:

Weekly Chair Yoga Practice Planner

Day 1:

Warm-Up:
Gentle neck stretches (2 minutes)
Shoulder rolls (1 minute)
Main Practice:
Basic seated poses (10 minutes)
Breathing exercises (3 minutes)
Cool-Down:
Seated forward fold (2 minutes)
Relaxation pose (5 minutes)
Day 2:

Warm-Up:
Arm circles (2 minutes)
Wrist stretches (1 minute)
Main Practice:
Gentle twists (8 minutes)
Modified sun salutations (5 minutes)
Cool-Down:
Seated side stretch (2 minutes)
Final relaxation (5 minutes)
Day 3:

Warm-Up:
Seated marches (2 minutes)
Ankle circles (1 minute)
Main Practice:
Chair squats (10 minutes)
Chair-supported warrior poses (5 minutes)
Cool-Down:
Seated spinal twist (2 minutes)
Deep breathing (3 minutes)
Day 4:

Warm-Up:

Seated cat-cow stretches (3 minutes)
Pelvic tilts (2 minutes)
Main Practice:
Seated mountain pose variations (8 minutes)
Chair-supported backbends (5 minutes)
Cool-Down:
Seated hip stretch (2 minutes)
Guided relaxation (5 minutes)
Day 5:

Warm-Up:
Gentle side-to-side bends (2 minutes)
Knee lifts (1 minute)
Main Practice:
Chair-supported balance exercises (10 minutes)
Seated meditation (5 minutes)
Cool-Down:
Seated heart opener (2 minutes)
Deep relaxation (5 minutes)
Tips for Using the Planner:
Personalize: Modify exercises and durations based on your comfort level and needs.
Progression: Gradually increase the intensity or duration of poses as your strength and flexibility improve.
Consistency: Aim for regular practice to experience the full benefits of chair yoga.
Variety: Include a mix of stretches, strengthening poses, and relaxation techniques in each session.
This planner provides a structured approach to planning chair yoga sessions, offering flexibility to adapt exercises and durations based on individual preferences and progress.

Appendix C: Detailed Pose Instructions

Step-by-Step Guides with Illustrations
Seated Mountain Pose

1. Starting Position:

Sit tall on a sturdy chair with feet flat on the floor, hip-width
apart.
Place hands on thighs, palms down, fingers spread wide.
2. Alignment:

Align your head over your shoulders, shoulders over hips.
Engage your core muscles and relax your shoulders down.
3. Inhale:

On an inhale, reach arms overhead, palms facing each other.
Keep shoulders relaxed and away from ears.
4. Exhale:

Exhale and press feet firmly into the floor.
Maintain a gentle lift through the spine and lengthen upward.
5. Hold:

Hold the pose for 5-10 breaths, maintaining steady breathing.
Feel the stretch through your sides and lengthening of the
spine.
6. Release:

To release, exhale and lower arms back to thighs.
Relax shoulders and take a moment to notice any changes in
your body.

How often should I practice chair yoga to see noticeable
benefits?

Consistency is key when practicing chair yoga. Aim for at least 2-3 sessions per week initially, gradually increasing as you become more comfortable. Regular practice helps reinforce muscle memory, improves flexibility, and enhances overall well-being. Some benefits, like improved flexibility and reduced stress, can be noticeable with consistent practice over a few weeks.

Can I combine chair yoga with other forms of exercise or yoga practices?

Chair yoga can complement other forms of exercise or yoga practices depending on your fitness level and goals. It's versatile enough to be integrated with gentle cardio exercises, resistance training, or even traditional mat-based yoga. Ensure that any additional exercises or practices are compatible with your health and fitness needs, and consult with a healthcare provider or fitness instructor for personalized advice.

Are there specific precautions I should take if I have existing health conditions?

Yes, if you have existing health conditions such as cardiovascular issues, joint problems, or chronic pain, it's crucial to consult with your healthcare provider before starting chair yoga. They can provide specific guidelines and modifications tailored to your condition to ensure safety and prevent exacerbation of symptoms. Always listen to your body during practice and modify poses as needed.

What should I do if I experience discomfort or pain during a pose?

Discomfort during chair yoga poses is common, especially if you're new to the practice or have physical limitations. If you experience sharp pain, stop the pose immediately and gently come back to a comfortable position. Modify the pose by reducing the range of motion or using props for support. If discomfort persists or worsens, consult a qualified yoga instructor or healthcare professional for guidance.

How can I progress from beginner to intermediate or advanced chair yoga practices?

Progression in chair yoga involves gradually increasing the complexity and intensity of poses as your strength and flexibility improve. Start with basic poses and gradually incorporate more challenging variations or sequences. Attend classes or workshops led by experienced instructors who can guide you through progressive stages safely. Focus on proper alignment and breath awareness to advance your practice effectively.

Are there certifications or qualifications for becoming a chair yoga instructor?

Yes, becoming a certified chair yoga instructor typically requires completing a specialized training program accredited by a recognized yoga alliance or association. These programs cover chair yoga techniques, anatomy, teaching methodology, and adapting practices for diverse populations, including seniors and individuals with disabilities. Certification ensures that instructors have the knowledge and skills to teach chair yoga safely and effectively.

How can I find local chair yoga classes or groups for seniors in my area?

To find local chair yoga classes, check community centers, senior centers, yoga studios, or fitness clubs in your area. Many offer specialized classes for seniors or those with mobility limitations. Online directories, social media groups, or local newspapers may also list classes. Contact instructors or organizers to inquire about class schedules, accessibility, and suitability for your needs.

Are there online resources or communities where I can connect with other chair yoga practitioners?

Yes, online resources such as forums, social media groups, and yoga websites often have communities dedicated to chair yoga practitioners. These platforms provide opportunities to share experiences, ask questions, and access additional resources like video tutorials, articles, and workshops. Engaging with online communities can offer support, motivation, and ongoing learning opportunities for chair yoga enthusiasts.

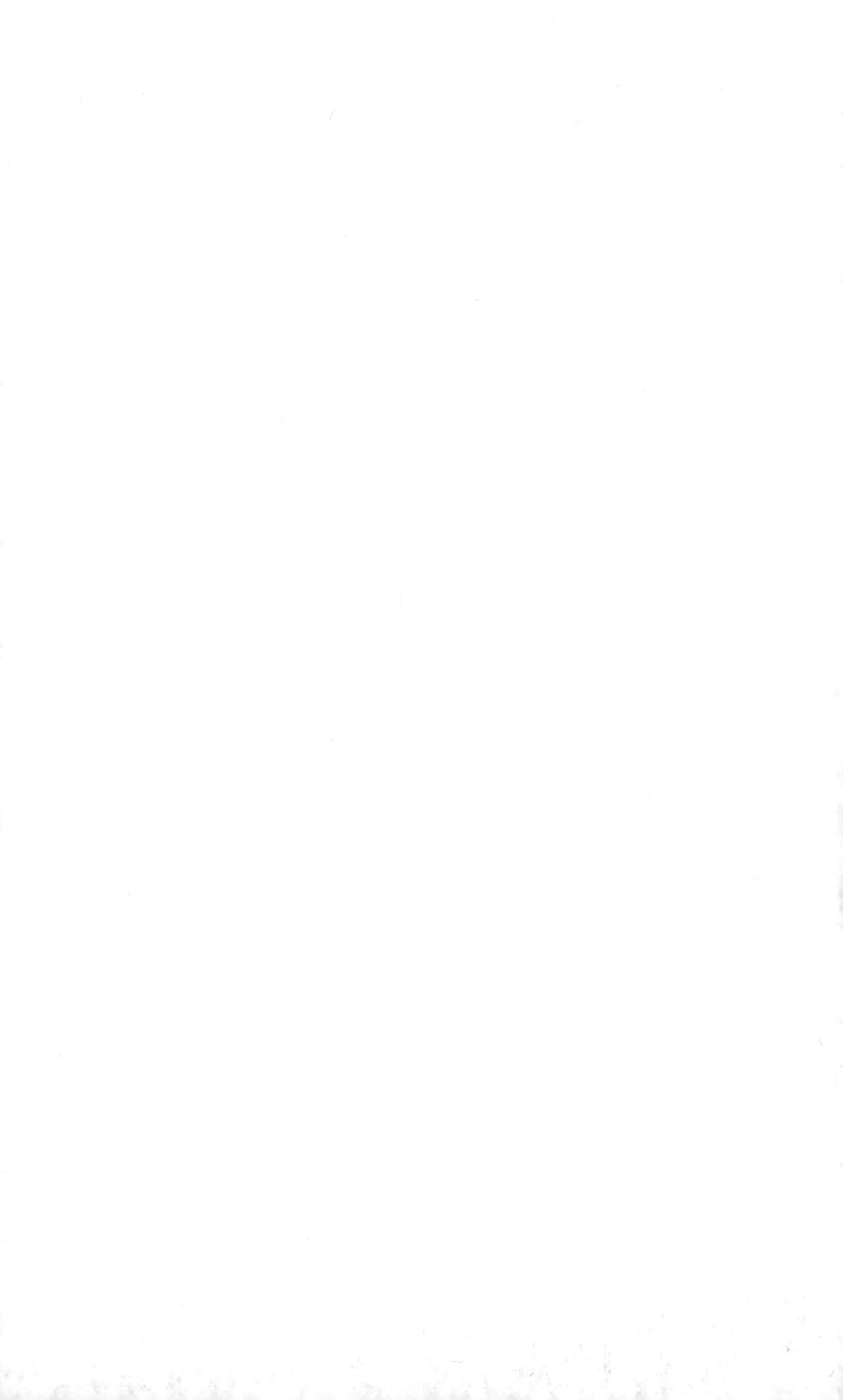